T0334696

Cambridge Elements ⎓

Elements in High-Risk Pregnancy: Management Options
edited by
David James
University of Nottingham
Philip Steer
Imperial College London
Carl Weiner
Creighton University School of Medicine
Stephen Robson
Newcastle University

SPONTANEOUS PRETERM LABOUR AND BIRTH (INCLUDING PRETERM PRE-LABOUR RUPTURE OF MEMBRANES)

Natasha L. Hezelgrave
Kings College London

Andrew H. Shennan
Kings College London

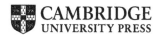

CAMBRIDGE
UNIVERSITY PRESS

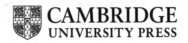

Shaftesbury Road, Cambridge CB2 8EA, United Kingdom

One Liberty Plaza, 20th Floor, New York, NY 10006, USA

477 Williamstown Road, Port Melbourne, VIC 3207, Australia

314–321, 3rd Floor, Plot 3, Splendor Forum, Jasola District Centre,
New Delhi – 110025, India

103 Penang Road, #05–06/07, Visioncrest Commercial, Singapore 238467

Cambridge University Press is part of Cambridge University Press & Assessment,
a department of the University of Cambridge.

We share the University's mission to contribute to society through the pursuit of
education, learning and research at the highest international levels of excellence.

www.cambridge.org
Information on this title: www.cambridge.org/9781009508919

DOI: 10.1017/9781009508940

First published 2025

A catalogue record for this publication is available from the British Library

ISBN 978-1-009-50891-9 Paperback
ISSN 2976-8330 (online)
ISSN 2976-8322 (print)

Additional resources for this publication at www.cambridge.org/hezelgrave-shennan

Spontaneous Preterm Labour and Birth (Including Preterm Pre-labour Rupture of Membranes)

Elements in High-Risk Pregnancy: Management Options

DOI: 10.1017/9781009508940
First published online: January 2025

Natasha L. Hezelgrave
Kings College London

Andrew H. Shennan
Kings College London

Author for correspondence: Natasha L. Hezelgrave,
natasha.hezelgrave@nhs.net

Abstract: Spontaneous preterm birth remains the leading cause of neonatal death, and the second leading cause of mortality worldwide in children below five years of age. The causes of preterm birth are multifactorial, likely contributing to why significant progress in reducing the incidence has been slow. This Element contains the most up-to-date evidence regarding the aetiology, epidemiology, and management of pregnancies at risk of, or complicated by, spontaneous preterm birth and preterm pre-labour rupture of membranes. It concentrates largely on those aspects potentially amenable to preventative intervention (i.e. cervical dysfunction and premature uterine contractility), as well as strategies to improve outcomes for infants born prematurely.

Keywords: birth, neonatal, pregnancy, preterm birth, preterm labour

ISBNs: 9781009508919 (PB), 9781009508940 (OC)
ISSNs: 2976-8330 (online), 2976-8322 (print)

Contents

An online appendix for this publication can be accessed at www.cambridge.org/hezelgrave-shennan

Commentary

Despite the long-standing focus on its prevention, spontaneous preterm birth (sPTB) remains the leading cause of neonatal death, and the second leading cause of mortality worldwide in children below five years of age, after pneumonia. Of those babies who survive, many have severe long-term physical and neurodevelopmental morbidity. A central problem is that the causes of preterm birth are multifactorial. About a third of preterm births are iatrogenic – that is, the baby is delivered electively because of maternal disease such as hypertension, or concerns about fetal well-being (e.g. fetal growth restriction). The causes of sPTB are equally varied, and include infection/inflammation, uterine distension (e.g. multiple pregnancy), antepartum haemorrhage, cervical dysfunction, and social factors. This Element will deal with sPTB (including preterm pre-labour rupture of membranes), concentrating on those aspects potentially amendable to preventative intervention (i.e. cervical dysfunction and premature uterine contractility).

The key to improving fetal outcomes for those at risk of sPTB are: first, the accurate prediction of preterm birth (using history, cervical length assessment using transvaginal ultrasonography, and biochemical tests of cervicovaginal mucus); second, the prevention of preterm birth using cervical cerclage or vaginal progesterone in selected cases; and, third, optimisation of outcomes for women with threatened preterm birth, including delaying delivery using tocolysis, administering antenatal therapy such as corticosteroids and magnesium sulphate for fetal lung development and neuroprotection, respectively, and ensuring appropriate place of birth, particularly important for those infants born at the extremes of viable gestation. Given that most women who present with preterm contractions do not go on to deliver preterm infants, the challenge is to accurately identify the appropriate recipients of these therapies, which do have some unwanted side effects. The balance of benefit is entirely negative if they are given to women who go on to deliver at term because the diagnosis of preterm labour (PTL) was incorrect. In this context, transvaginal ultrasound and fetal fibronectin testing are useful tools to assess risk and guide care. Preterm pre-labour rupture of membranes, in particular, requires careful balancing of clinical decision-making between optimising gestation of delivery for the infant and avoiding maternal or fetal infective morbidity. This involves monitoring closely for signs of chorioamnionitis, which, if diagnosed, necessitate urgent delivery. Current research strategies are focussed on in-depth understanding and individual phenotyping of the pathophysiology behind sPTB, in order to improve strategies to identify those at risk and prevent preterm birth.

Definitions and Epidemiology

Preterm labour is defined by the World Health Organization (WHO) as the onset of labour before 37 completed weeks or 259 days' gestation, and after the gestation of viability (this can be 22–8 weeks depending on definition and setting).[1] *Preterm birth* (PTB) is the birth of an infant before 37 completed weeks' gestation. Spontaneous PTB (sPTB) encompasses spontaneous onset of uterine contractions resulting in delivery, or preterm pre-labour rupture of membranes (PPROM), which is spontaneous rupture of the membranes before 37 completed weeks' gestation and before the onset of contractions. Spontaneous PTB accounts for approximately 70% of all preterm deliveries.[2] The remaining 30% are iatrogenic (physician-initiated for maternal or fetal health indications). Of sPTBs, just over 60% result from spontaneous onset of contractions, and the remainder follow PPROM.[3] Only spontaneous prematurity will be considered for this Element review.

The gestational endpoint of 37 completed weeks (i.e. 37^{+0}) was defined by the WHO as the beginning of 'term' from a statistical analysis of the distribution of gestation of birth based on the first day of the last menstrual period.[4] However, in terms of functional outcome, measured according to need for special care, while continued functional improvement in the newborn occurs up to the due date (e.g. babies born in the early term period at 37–8 weeks have more problems than those born at 39–40 weeks),[5] the major improvement occurs at 34–7 weeks' gestation in high-income settings, and there is a progressive rise in morbidity and mortality rates the further from term that birth occurs.

Internationally, the following PTB categories are recognised by the WHO: extremely preterm (<28 weeks), very preterm (28–32 weeks), and moderate to late preterm (32–7 weeks).[1] Moderate and late PTB can be further split to emphasise late prematurity (34 to under 37 completed weeks) in contrast to moderate prematurity (32–3 completed weeks).[6] Notably, even babies born at 37–8 weeks have higher adverse outcome risks than those born at 39–40 weeks,[7] although this may be related to the reason for delivery. Thus, being 'born early' should be seen as a continuum rather than as an 'all-or-nothing' phenomenon.

Despite the long-term focus on its prevention, sPTB (resulting from PTL or PPROM) remains the leading cause of neonatal death, and the second leading cause of under-5 mortality, after pneumonia, worldwide. While reliable global data are difficult to obtain, in 2010, an estimated 11.1% of all live births globally were preterm,[8] representing 15 million births <37 weeks' gestation and responsible for over 1 million neonatal deaths per year.[6] It may also contribute to at least 50% of neonatal deaths worldwide, as a risk factor for other causes of neonatal death (e.g. infection).[9] Globally, the incidence of PTB ranges from 5 to 18% with the greatest burden in developing countries. Worryingly, the incidence of PTB is thought to be increasing in all regions with reliable data.[8,10]

Pathophysiology

Preterm birth is a complex health problem, with demographic, clinical, and behavioural determinants of individual risk. While the precise mechanisms are unknown, PTL may be initiated by a number of different factors with distinct biological pathways. These include inflammation and infection (e.g. clinical/subclinical chorioamnionitis, ascending genital tract infection, bacteriuria, and maternal systemic infection),[11,12,13] steroid hormone (including progesterone) imbalance, uterine distension (including multiple pregnancy and polyhydramnios), cervical insufficiency, and placental vascular causes, culminating in a common clinical scenario: cervical ripening, uterine contractions, and early birth.[14] Precursors vary by gestational age,[4] (85% of sPTB <28 weeks have evidence of subclinical chorioamnionitis) and by demographic and environmental factors, modulated by genetic factors[15,16,17,18,19] although the cause remains undetermined in up to half of all cases.

Consequences of PTB

Fetal/Neonatal

The health consequences for a baby born preterm are far-reaching, particularly for infants born at <32 weeks' gestation (Figure 1). Gestational age is highly related to outcome, both mortality and morbidity. The series of EPICure studies examined short- and longer-term health outcomes of infants born between 20 and 26 weeks' gestation in the UK and Ireland in 1995 and 2006 and demonstrated increased survival and lower rates of disability with each additional week of gestation.[20,21] Infants born at 23, 24, and 25 weeks' gestation in 2006 had 19, 40, and 66% survival to discharge from hospital respectively (as a proportion of all live births). Major morbidities associated with extreme prematurity include respiratory distress syndrome (RDS), necrotising enterocolitis (NEC), retinopathy of prematurity, and major cerebral injury (including intraventricular haemorrhage). Longer-term problems include cerebral palsy, neurodevelopmental delay, deafness, visual impairment, and chronic lung disease. The prevalence of long-term disability (neurodevelopmental impairment) is also negatively correlated with the length of gestation.

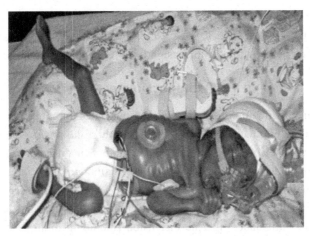

Figure 1 Preterm infant born at 23 weeks' gestation.
Reproduced by kind permission of the mother.

Maternal

Much of the maternal risk associated with prematurity is derived from the inherent maternal pathology that precedes the birth, including preeclampsia, antepartum haemorrhage and maternal infection. These may precipitate PTB or necessitate iatrogenic delivery of the fetus by induction of labour or caesarean section, which also carry their own risks for the mother. In particular, caesarean section of a very preterm infant carries a risk of significant maternal morbidity related to a poorly formed lower uterine segment. Other maternal risks include the complications of prophylactic interventions to reduce the risk of sPTB (see later).

The psychological impact of premature birth on a woman, her partner, and her family can be substantial. Threatened PTB frequently involves a protracted hospital stay. This can involve geographic dislocation according to availability of neonatal cots. There is tremendous anxiety and uncertainty regarding timing of delivery and likely outcome. Extremely preterm infants have high mortality and morbidity rates, often involving care in a high-dependency neonatal unit with accompanied emotional upheaval and delayed maternal–infant bonding. The longer-term emotional, physical, and social consequences of caring for an infant with long-term chronic physical and developmental needs are difficult to quantify. Apart from the profound impact on the children and their families, additional consequences of PTB are the enormous economic consequences for health services.[22,23]

Clinical Risk Factors for PTB

There are a number of recognised modifiable and unmodifiable maternal pre-pregnancy risk factors for prematurity, the most significant and consistently identified being a woman's history of previous sPTB, with a recurrence risk of approximately 15%[24] and potentially higher when the previous PTB was <28 weeks,[25] or there has been more than one previous PTB.[26]

Invasive cervical surgery (including laser and cold knife conisation and loop electrosurgical excision procedures (LEEP)) performed for treatment of cervical intraepithelial neoplasia (CIN) is a risk factor for mid-trimester miscarriage, PPROM, and PTB.[27] Furthermore, damage to the cervix, not only after excision procedures, but also during caesarean section, particularly when performed at full dilatation, may also confer increased risk of sPTB.[28,29,30]

Müllerian duct abnormalities are associated with risk of prematurity,[31] as are various social, demographic and behavioural risk factors including extremes of maternal age, a short interpregnancy interval, low pre-pregnancy body mass index (BMI) and poor weight gain in pregnancy, low socioeconomic status, maternal smoking and drug use.[32,33] In the UK and USA, women of black African, African-American and Afro-Caribbean ethnic origin are consistently reported to be at higher risk of PTB than women of white European origin.[2] The biological basis of these risk factors is poorly understood, but persist even after correction for known PTB risk factors such as smoking, maternal education, and socioeconomic status. Biological risk factors such as the higher incidence of urogenital infection in black women (particularly bacterial vaginosis (BV)) are likely to contribute, as well as underlying genetic factors.[34] Healthcare also plays a significant role. There is little robust data on the effect of sexual intercourse during pregnancy, and observational studies are hindered by confounding factors (e.g. age, socioeconomic factors, avoidance of sexual intercourse in women at risk). In general, the data are reassuring that intercourse during pregnancy is not associated with PTB. However, in clinical practice, in the presence of a very short cervix (bulging membranes or diagnosed via transvaginal ultrasound scan), the authors do frequently advise women to abstain from intercourse, in order to avoid introduction of infection or disruption of precarious membranes. Risk factors for PPROM are largely similar to those related to preterm spontaneous labour with intact membranes, but infection is thought to play a particularly significant role.

Management Options for sPTB and PPROM

Pre-pregnancy

Women at risk of sPTB and/or PPROM (see earlier) should be offered pre-pregnancy counselling. The risk of recurrence in future pregnancy and the possible options should be discussed. In addition, advice about cessation of smoking, alcohol intake, recreational drug use, and optimisation of weight should be included.

Prenatal

Prediction of PTB/PPROM

Current attempts to prevent PTB (spontaneous onset or PPROM) rely on identifying women at increased risk of PTB from their history and clinical examination, and screening them using tests such as ultrasound cervical length (CL) and fibronectin measurement in vaginal fluid. Depending on the findings (or sometimes on the history alone), interventions such as cervical cerclage, progesterone therapy, or a cervical pessary while the woman is still asymptomatic are then recommended. Both transvaginal CL and cervical fluid biomarkers, such as fetal fibronectin (fFN) and phosphorylated insulin-like growth factor binding protein, are increasingly recognised as being useful for the prediction of PTB in both symptomatic and asymptomatic women. Given the paucity of proven interventions to prevent prematurity, it is logical that high-risk surveillance and screening is targeted to the population in which preventive intervention has been shown to be beneficial: in particular, those with previous premature birth or mid-trimester miscarriage. In practice, women with other risk factors, including extensive cervical surgery, uterine abnormalities, and previous caesarean at full dilatation, may also be referred for screening (see the guidelines in the Online Appendix), although the value of established prophylactic interventions has not yet been demonstrated in these populations.

Cervical Screening by Transvaginal Ultrasonography

The process of labour is associated with progressive cervical shortening, effacement, and dilatation. Effacement and shortening ('funnelling') usually begins at the internal cervical os and can be demonstrated using transvaginal ultrasonography well before dilatation of the external os can be detected on digital vaginal examination. In pregnancies destined to reach term, this gradual process usually begins sometime after 32 weeks' gestation but may not occur until immediately before delivery. Measurement of CL between 14 and 24 weeks has been shown to be a sensitive predictor of sPTB in both low- and high-risk pregnancies (the

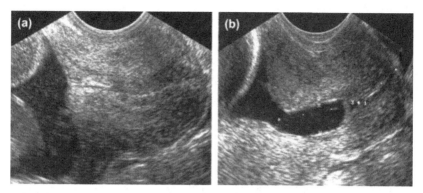

Figure 2 Transvaginal ultrasound of (a) a normal cervix, and (b) a short cervix with funnelling. Reprinted from Simcox, R, Shennan, A. Cervical cerclage in the prevention of preterm birth. Best Pract Res Clin Obstet Gynaecol 2007; 21: 831–42, with permission from Elsevier.

risk of prematurity is inversely related to the CL: the shorter it is, the higher the risk), and thus is the most commonly recommended screening tool to identify pregnancies at higher risk of PTB and those who may benefit from prophylactic intervention.

Cervical length measured by transvaginal ultrasonography in a general obstetric (low-risk) population has a Gaussian distribution; the mean length at 23 weeks' gestation is 35–8 mm, with the 5th percentile at approximately 23 mm.[35,36] A standardised technique for measurement of the cervix using transvaginal ultrasonography has been described.[37] Several studies have demonstrated that risk of preterm delivery is substantially greater in high-risk women with CL <25 mm (approximately the 10th centile) between 14 and 24 weeks' gestation, and that this risk increases exponentially with decreasing CL.[38,39,40] Figure 2 illustrates a normal cervix compared with a short cervix which demonstrates funnelling.

A short cervix is predictive of PTB even in women without a previous history of PTB (over half of PTBs occur in such women),[35,36] as well as in those who have risk factors for PTB. However, given the low prevalence of a short cervix and PTB in the general population, the number needed to screen to identify one short cervix is very high. Furthermore, there is little evidence at present to support a program of low-risk screening using CL because an effective intervention to improve pregnancy outcome in these women has not been demonstrated. Thus, most guidelines (Online Appendix) recommend serial cervical surveillance (usually between 16 and 24 weeks) only for those women with a risk factor for PTB, the most common being previous PTB although screening of women with other risk factors such as cervical surgery, uterine anomaly or previous full dilation cesarian section is increasingly common. Cervical length measurement is also predictive of sPTB in women with multiple pregnancies,[41] although the problem remains that, as with low-risk singleton pregnancies, there are currently no proven interventions to prevent PTB or improve outcome in asymptomatic women with multiple pregnancies.

Fetal Fibronectin

Fetal fibronectin is a glycoprotein found in placental tissue, in amniotic fluid, and between the chorion and decidua, normally detectable in the cervicovaginal fluid (CVF) in pregnancy before the fusion of the decidua and fetal membranes. CVF fFN concentrations drop and may become undetectable from 18 weeks' gestation. After this time, release of fFN into the CVF by presumed inflammatory, infective, or mechanical disruption to the choriodecidual interface is associated with an increased risk of premature delivery, which can be detected using a rapid bedside test. Arguably most valuable as a 'rule-out' test, a negative fFN (<50 ng/ml) detected at 24–26 weeks' gestation has a negative predictive value (NPV) for PTB (proportion of women who test negative and deliver at term) of 96%.[42] However, the positive predictive value (PPV; proportion of women identified as positive who actually deliver preterm) is relatively low (<30%) at clinically important gestations, which limits the utility of the test. More recently, a quantitative bedside fFN test has been developed, and studies have demonstrated enhanced prediction compared with the traditional qualitative (positive/negative) test in both symptomatic and asymptomatic women. fFN concentration correlates directly with the subsequent incidence of sPTB. For symptomatic and asymptomatic women, use of alternative incremental thresholds (10 and 50, and 200 and 500 ng/ml, respectively) enhances PPV for early delivery (an improved 'rule-in' test) within 14 days and before 34 weeks, while the NPV remains high at every threshold.[43,44] This allows clinicians to stratify individual patient risk more accurately and tailor management accordingly. A threshold of 10 ng/ml has sufficiently high sensitivity and NPV to determine which high-risk women are unlikely to deliver preterm. In contrast, the higher the CVF quantitative fFN concentration, the greater the need for surveillance and therapeutic intervention. Further research is required to evaluate how quantitative fFN may be used to identify asymptomatic women who would benefit from prophylactic intervention, but it is increasingly used (often alongside transvaginal ultrasound CL screening) to risk stratify women at risk of PTB.

Prevention of PTB

Detection and Treatment of Infection

An inflammatory cascade, often with an associated bacterial infection, is implicated in up to 40% of sPTB, and in reality, it may be even higher, given the limitations of current culture-based identification techniques. While we do not yet have reliable clinical tools to detect or treat most of these infections, the detection and treatment of bacterial vaginosis (BV) and asymptomatic bacteriuria may still have a role in prevention of PTB.

BV is an imbalance of vaginal flora, characterised by an increase in mixed anaerobic flora and a reduction in the proportion of lactobacillus bacteria. While often asymptomatic, BV can manifest as a grey discoloured vaginal discharge, with a characteristic 'fishy' odour. Typically diagnosed using Amsel's criteria[45] use of a Gram stain of a vaginal swab is an accepted alternative method. BV in pregnancy has consistently been demonstrated to be associated with poor perinatal outcome, most commonly an increased risk of prematurity.[46,47] Results of trials of treatment of BV in pregnancy, however, have not been encouraging. The largest meta-analysis[47] showed antibiotic therapy to be effective at eradicating BV and restoring normal vaginal flora when compared with placebo/no treatment, but there was no observed reduction in the rate of premature delivery before 32-, 34-, or 37-weeks' gestation, nor were there any differences in neonatal outcome. Although there was a significant reduction in late miscarriage in women with BV treated with antibiotics compared with placebo/no treatment (RR: 0.20; 95% CI: 0.05–0.76; two trials, 1,270 women), worryingly, in several of the smaller trials, there were worse outcomes in high-risk women treated with antibiotics compared with placebo.[48,49,50] Thus, there is little evidence currently to support the routine screening of low-risk women for BV, with some evidence that treating women at 'high risk' based on the presence of BV may cause harm. Even when treating women at high risk of prematurity for other reasons, more evidence is needed before routine screening could be recommended. Nonetheless, given the observed reduction (although in only two trials) of late miscarriage in women with BV treated with clindamycin before 20 weeks, further study is warranted in this area. Treatment of symptomatic BV (as opposed to BV diagnosed only by routine screening) is still clinically appropriate.

Asymptomatic bacteriuria (the presence of bacteria in the urine without clinical symptoms) complicates 2–10% of all pregnancies,[51] and nitrite dipstick testing of urine as a screening test at each antenatal visit is commonly recommended to trigger, if positive, culture of a midstream specimen followed by antibiotic treatment of confirmed bacteriuria, thereby to reduce the incidence of pyelonephritis in the mother. However, there is conflicting evidence about the benefits of antibiotic treatment for asymptomatic bacteriuria in relation to the prevention of PTB. Villar *et al.* found that antibiotic treatment for asymptomatic bacteriuria reduced the incidence of spontaneous early delivery and low birth weight which persisted when only the three trials which reported the outcome of PTB <37 weeks' gestation were included in the analysis.[52] However, this finding was not replicated by a 2007 Cochrane meta-analysis of 14 randomised controlled trials (RCTs), showing that antibiotic treatment was associated with a reduction in the incidence of low-birth-weight babies but not prematurity.[53]

About 22–35% of women carry Group B streptococci (GBS; *Streptococcus agalactiae*) in their gut and lower vagina. There is some evidence that maternal GBS colonisation is associated with an increased risk of PTB[54] especially where there is evidence of ascending infection (bacteriuria). However there is no evidence that carriage can be eradicated (as opposed to reducing bacterial load) with antibiotic therapy and therefore antibiotic administration is only indicated if there is evidence of active infection (e.g. in the urinary tract).

Cervical Cerclage

The placement of a suture around the cervix is a common obstetric procedure performed in women at high risk of mid-trimester miscarriage or PTB, despite the lack of a well-defined population for whom there is clear evidence of benefit. The mechanism of action is not clearly understood; it is likely that cervical cerclage may provide structural strength to a shortening or weak cervix, but it is also likely to assist in protecting from ascending pathogens by maintaining a mucus plug in the cervix, thereby creating a biochemical and/or immunological barrier. The role (and success) of a cerclage may be dependent on the underlying pathophysiology of prematurity, and this is yet to be clearly elucidated.

Evidence for the benefit of cerclage is largely derived from meta-analysis of underpowered RCTs, many of which lack relevant clinical endpoints. The women in whom cerclage may be indicated can be broadly divided into three groups: those who have suffered multiple recurrent pregnancy loss (history-indicated cerclage); those found to have a short cervix on ultrasound scan with a prior history of spontaneous early delivery (ultrasound-indicated cerclage); and those with painless cervical dilatation resulting in bulging fetal membranes ('rescue cerclage').

History-Indicated Cerclage

Placement of a cervical cerclage in early pregnancy in women with previous mid-trimester fetal loss or sPTB is common obstetric practice. This practice has been evaluated in a number of trials, the largest of which was the Medical Research Council/Royal College of Obstetricians and Gynaecologists (MRC/RCOG) randomised trial that included 1,299 patients and was published in 1993.[55] This trial did not demonstrate benefit of suture placement to reduce PTB <37 weeks or improve neonatal outcome overall but did demonstrate a small reduction in risk of early PTB (<33 weeks), particularly in the small number of women (107) with a history of three or more pregnancies ending before 37 weeks' gestation, when the risk was reduced by half. The February 2022 UK RCOG Green-top guideline number 75[56] advises that a history-indicated suture should be placed in women with three or more previous PTBs and/or second-trimester losses. In practice, this is usually done after an early scan, at around 12–15 weeks. This is not recommended by the 2014 American College of Obstetricians and Gynecologists (ACOG) guidelines, who restrict cerclage recommendations to those women with a short cervix.[57] It is important to discuss the risks and benefits of such a procedure for eligible women, including the uncertainty surrounding the small evidence base, to allow fully informed patient-led decision-making. Furthermore, despite a lack of evidence for benefit, women with fewer than three previous premature deliveries may elect to have a prophylactic suture placed as an alternative to cervical surveillance, and this decision-making is supported by the recent UK Saving Babies Lives Version 2 guideline.

Ultrasound-Indicated Cerclage

Ultrasound-indicated cerclage is the placement of cervical cerclage in women who have cervical shortening on transvaginal ultrasound scan (usually <25 mm). While not shown to reduce the incidence of PTB in women with a short cervix but no other risk factors for prematurity (likely due to lack of power given low PTB rates in this population),[58,59] in women who have experienced a prior preterm delivery, there is stronger evidence for the benefit of cerclage insertion. Meta-analysis of four RCTs confirmed that in women with a previous second-trimester miscarriage between 16- and 23-weeks' gestation, or PTB before 37 weeks, cerclage significantly reduced delivery before 35 weeks in women who developed a short cervix by approximately 50%.[59] On this evidence, it is reasonable to offer ultrasound surveillance of all women with a prior PTB before 34 weeks, or a mid-trimester loss, and to offer cerclage if the cervix is <25 mm before 24 weeks' gestation. The role of cerclage in women without a prior history remains unclear, although it may be offered as part of individualised care following a discussion of relevant risks and benefits.

Emergency Cerclage with Exposed Fetal Membranes ('Rescue Cerclage')

As the cervix prematurely shortens prior to an early birth, the membranes around the fetus may prolapse through the internal and external cervical os, so that on clinical presentation the fetal membranes can be visualised herniating through the cervical canal on ultrasound or speculum examination. Women can present asymptomatically as part of routine CL screening, particularly <24 weeks' gestation, or present symptomatically with pain, a feeling of pressure in the vagina, or watery vaginal loss, probably related to a transudate across the exposed membrane, often thought (incorrectly) to be ruptured membranes. While, in general, pregnancies presenting before fetal viability with bulging fetal membranes have a very poor prognosis, a rescue cerclage may be placed after reducing the membranes with the aim to re-seal the cervix, preventing further membrane herniation. Deep Trendelenberg position is required for the procedure, and a Foley catheter balloon or a Lee tube can be used to retract the membranes back into the uterine cavity, after which the cervix is closed with a purse-string suture. Only one small RCT has been performed to compare cerclage (and intraoperative indomethacin) with expectant management, and this only included 23 women (16 singleton and seven twin pregnancies) with bulging fetal membranes at a mean gestation of 22–3 weeks.[60] Women in the cerclage group stayed pregnant longer and delivered later (29.9 vs 25.9 weeks), with a reduction in sPTB before 34 weeks' gestation (53 vs 100%; $p = 0.02$) and significant reduction in composite neonatal morbidity.

Given that infection and inflammation may contribute to the process of cervical shortening, which increases the exposure of fetal membranes to vaginal microorganisms, there are concerns that insertion of a stitch may exacerbate further inflammation and infection. Moreover, the membranes can be ruptured inadvertently during the procedure. This may result in delivery at a lower gestation than with expectant management, or the survival of a more mature but more damaged baby by virtue of chorioamnionitis, neonatal sepsis, and associated fetal inflammatory brain injury, thus inadvertently increasing overall morbidity.[61] There is insufficient evidence to recommend routine amniocentesis or genital tract screening prior to cerclage, as there are no clear data demonstrating that it improves outcome. Currently, clinical practice in this area is extremely heterogeneous and further research is vital to address this question. Ongoing RCTs in the UK are in progress to gain further insight into the risks and benefits of emergency cerclage. Until these results are available, judicious use of cerclage should be applied in selected cases, after careful counselling, can be recommended. It seems plausible that the success of the procedure depends upon the experience and skill of the operator performing the cerclage.

Cerclage Technique

There is little consensus about the optimal technique for cervical cerclage insertion. A low transvaginal cerclage is often a suture inserted in a 'purse-string' fashion (sometimes known as a McDonald suture), placed at the cervicovaginal junction, without surgical mobilisation of the bladder (Figure 3). Performed under spinal anaesthetic, it can usually be removed without anaesthetic. A high vaginal suture (sometimes referred to as Shirodkar suture) places the stitch at the level of the cardinal ligaments by mobilising the bladder upwards. The knot is frequently buried, requiring regional anaesthesia for removal. There are numerous modifications of these techniques, depending on individual preference and experience. This makes direct comparison difficult, but a secondary analysis of four RCTs comparing McDonald and Shirodkar cerclage in women with a CL of <15 mm demonstrated no difference in prematurity before 33 weeks' gestation,[62] and so, unless it

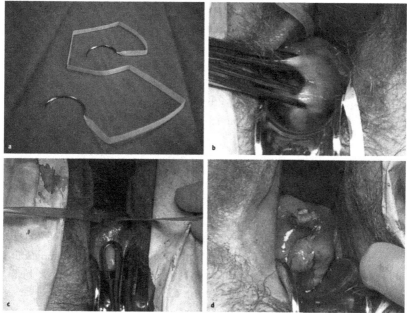

Figure 3 Insertion of a purse-string (McDonald) cervical suture, using (a) Mersilene tape. (b) Sponge forceps are used to grasp the cervix and the suture is inserted from the 12 o'clock to the 3 o'clock position and continued clockwise with four 'bites' taken until the 12 o'clock position is reached. (c) An anterior knot is tied, and (d) a double knot facilitates removal. Reproduced from Chandirmani, M, Tribe, RM, Shennan, AH. Preterm labour and prematurity. Obstetrics, Gynaecology and Reproductive Medicine 2007; 17: 232–7, with permission from Elsevier.

is impossible to place a high McDonald suture due to cervical deficiency (particularly the anterior lip), a Shirodkar suture does not appear to confer an advantage.

Cervical cerclage may also be performed via the abdominal route, with the intention to place the suture high around the cervix, adjacent to the fetal membranes. This procedure is often performed after failed vaginal cerclage, or in patients with extensive surgery to the cervix (e.g. after trachelectomy). One RCT involving over 100 women who had suffered a preterm delivery <28 weeks' gestation despite vaginal cerclage placement (ultrasound-indicated or history-indicated)[63] demonstrated a significant reduction in births <32 weeks with abdominally inserted sutures, and reduced neonatal mortality compared to both high and low vaginal sutures. Abdominal sutures require delivery by caesarean section, with two laparotomies per pregnancy, and therefore should be reserved for women with failed vaginal cerclage or such deficiency of the cervix that a vaginal approach is impractical. Laparoscopic procedures can be performed, and appear to be equally efficacious. Pre-pregnancy cerclage is preferable and does not appear to impact on fertility or early pregnancy complications.

Finally, as infective morbidity is commonly associated with preterm risk, there is uncertainty about the optimum suture material for cerclage. An RCT reported in 2022 comparing monofilament with braided suture material demonstrated no difference in pregnancy loss between the randomised groups. More women with a monofilament suture experienced removal complications (including need for anaesthetic), but significantly fewer developed chorioamnionitis (4 vs 7%).[64]

Progesterone Therapy

Progesterone is a hormone responsible for maintaining uterine quiescence during pregnancy, and may modulate cytokine and contraction-associated protein expression and activity. In recent years, antenatal progesterone therapy has been advocated (falling in and out of favour as conflicting studies are published and meta-analyses updated) to prevent premature birth. Progesterone therapy typically consists of vaginal capsules/gel or pessaries (usually for women with a previous history of PTB and/or a short cervix on ultrasound scan, or intramuscular injection of 17-hydroxyprogesterone caproate (17-OHP) once weekly. However, the optimal route of administration, dose, agent, and timing are not known, nor the effects on long-term maternal or neonatal outcomes.

The most recent individual patient data (IPD) meta-analysis[65] of progestogens to prevent PTB showed a reduction in risk of PTB using both vaginal progesterone and 17-OHP for high-risk women (previous PTB or those with a short cervix). However, it is notable that the largest trials of these trials (>1,000 women with a history of PTB randomised to 17-OHP or placebo) showed no efficacy,[66] and the external validity and reproducibility of previous studies that demonstrated a large effect[67] have been questioned.[68,69,70] Included in this IPD meta-analysis was the only large trial of progesterone that showed significant benefit,[71] which has been criticised, including by the US Food and Drug Administration (FDA), for discrepancies in data between sites. The use of 17-OHP in the USA has now been withdrawn by the FDA due to non-efficacy and potential risks. For those women with a history of prematurity and a short CL, it would seem reasonable, therefore, to prescribe vaginal progesterone (while further evidence of safety and benefit to the baby is being sought), with associated counselling regarding likely safety but still unclear efficacy. In contrast, for all women with a history of PTB (regardless of CL), the most recent meta-analysis evaluating vaginal progesterone use in women with a history of PTB only showed no benefit from vaginal progesterone;[72] its use in these women, although a common clinical practice, should be avoided in the absence of further data to show benefit.

Four RCTs involving multiple pregnancies have reported no significant benefit from the use of vaginal progesterone (90–400 mg/day) regardless of CL to prevent PTB.[73,74,75,76] However, given that a short cervix is a predictor of prematurity for multiple pregnancies as well as singletons, it remains to be seen whether progesterone therapy confers benefit in multiple pregnancies in which cervical shortening occurs.[77]

Arabin Pessary

The Arabin pessary is a round flexible device that is designed to be inserted into the vagina in the upper vaginal fornix in order to support and incline the cervix with the intention of preventing preterm cervical shortening and premature birth. An RCT of treatment of a short cervix in singleton pregnancies showed promising results, namely, a reduction in sPTB of <34 weeks and improved neonatal outcome in women with a short cervix.[78] However, concerns have been raised about the generalisability of the study, given the very high PTB rate in the control group, and subsequent RCTs have demonstrated no benefit.[79,80] This was confirmed in a 2017 meta-analysis.[81] Nor does the pessary reduce PTB in multiple pregnancies.[82]

Diagnosis of True PTL

The onset of labour refers to regular uterine contractions (at least one every 10 minutes), associated with documented cervical change or rupture of fetal membranes. In the absence of cervical change or ruptured membranes, a clinical diagnosis of threatened PTL can be made. Most women diagnosed with threatened PTL do not go on to deliver preterm, therefore screening tests can also be used to identify which women are at the highest risk of delivering imminently, and who would potentially benefit from interventions to delay PTB and/or improve maternal and fetal outcomes.

Biochemical Tests

For women already symptomatic of PTL (but with cervical dilatation <3 cm), the qualitative fFN test (described earlier) has an NPV of > 96%, which prevents unnecessary admission and intervention for the majority of women who present with contractions but do not go on to deliver, though its PPV is more modest. As with asymptomatic screening, using the test quantitatively provides enhanced prediction. The combination of risk factors for PTB, fFN result, and CL has been assessed and validated in a prediction algorithm for both asymptomatic high-risk women (AUC: 0.76 for prediction of PTB < 34 weeks' gestation),[83] and women symptomatic of PTL (AUC: 0.92 for prediction of PTB within 2 weeks of presentation).[84] These have been combined into a free mobile phone application (QUiPP), which provides individualised risk scores for women based on their risk factors, gestation, fFN concentration, and CL measurement, now used widely in the UK. A cluster randomised trial of 1,872 women in South-East England found that the QUiPP app accurately identified those women at highest risk of delivery (ROC: 0.90), representing an accurate method to identify those likely to benefit most from PTL interventions.[85]

A number of other commercially available biochemical tests for prediction of PTB in symptomatic women are also available. Phosphorylated insulin-like growth factor binding protein 1 (phIGFBP-1), produced by the placental decidual cells, is released into the CVF after presumed tissue damage to the choriodecidual interface.[86] A qualitative test (positive/negative), it is measured from a speculum-obtained vaginal swab between 22 and 36 weeks' gestation, with a high NPV (95%) for spontaneous preterm delivery but with poor positive predictive value.[87] Placental α microglobulin-1 (PAMG-1) is a glycoprotein synthesised by the decidua, and found in high concentrations in the amniotic fluid, but with low levels in the CVF.[88] It is obtained using a vaginal swab inserted directly into the vagina, obviating the need for a speculum, and measured using bedside dipstick analysis. One small study ($n = 101$) has demonstrated 97% NPV and 78% PPV for delivery within seven days in symptomatic women, with similarly high predictive value for delivery within two weeks.[89] While clearly requiring evaluation in a larger group of women, this has promising short-term prediction potential, although prediction of delivery >14 days after testing is not clear. However, there is very little evidence for its use compared to CL and other biochemical markers.

CL Measurement

Transvaginal ultrasound assessment of CL has demonstrated value in assessing women who present with symptoms suggestive of PTL, though requirements for a trained operator and equipment limit frontline use, particularly for women presenting outside clinic hours. A prospective case cohort study demonstrated that for symptomatic women with a CL <15 mm at <32 weeks' gestation, the PPV for delivery within seven days was 47% (a more than five-fold higher risk of sPTB than women with CL measuring >15 mm).[90] While there is a paucity of RCTs to demonstrate that knowledge of CL reduces sPTB rate or improves fetal outcome, it is likely that early diagnosis of 'true' PTL enables better targeting of interventions such as maternal corticosteroid administration to enhance pulmonary maturity of the fetus, the infusion of magnesium sulphate as a neuroprotective agent, and in utero transfer to a more appropriate birth setting if necessary. Equally important, this avoids unnecessary overtreatment of women who are not destined to give birth preterm.

Diagnosis of Preterm PPROM

In the majority of women, the diagnosis of PPROM can be confirmed based on a suspicious history and unequivocal loss of amniotic fluid. However, in approximately 10% of cases, the diagnosis of rupture of membranes is difficult to establish. The patient's history, a sterile vaginal speculum examination, and an abdominal ultrasound are the first steps in achieving the diagnosis of PPROM. Ultrasound is used to measure the amniotic fluid index (AFI), the estimated fetal weight (EFW), the presenting part of the baby, and, if indicated, the biophysical profile. If not already performed at first- and second-trimester scans, determination of the correct gestational age and an extensive ultrasound scan looking for congenital abnormalities should be carried out. Digital vaginal examination should be avoided where possible to avoid introducing infection, unless the patient is suspected to be in labour; the performance of a digital vaginal examination is associated with a shorter interval between PPROM and delivery when compared to a sterile speculum examination.[91,92]

For many years, a combination of pooling of amniotic fluid during speculum examination, alkaline pH determination, and microscopic evidence of ferning was used to determine rupture of membranes. These tests are, however, more prone to false-positive results due to vaginal contamination with blood, urine, or semen.[93] Additional tests have been designed to aid in the diagnosis of rupture of membranes, especially in equivocal cases. Review articles list several candidates and find limited evidence to prefer one test over another.[94,95] One study shows a very good performance of insulin-like growth factor binding protein 1 (IGFB-1) when compared to the gold standard of intra-amniotic injection of indigo carmine,[96] though false-positive results have been described in cases of IGFB-1 detection in patients with PPROM who were also in labour.[97] Alternatively, PAMG-1 can assist in diagnosing PPROM in equivocal cases.[98]

Management of Threatened and Established PTL and Confirmed PPROM

Initial Assessment

When a woman presents with threatened or established PTL, a careful assessment of fetal and maternal condition must be performed. A detailed history followed by a vaginal speculum examination can establish whether membranes have ruptured, and the degree of cervical effacement and dilatation. In the absence of ruptured membranes, a biochemical test such as an fFN test (as previously described) can be performed to assess the risk of imminent and subsequent preterm delivery, and a transvaginal CL ultrasound can be performed. Given that most women who present with symptoms of PTL do not deliver preterm, this will help guide decisions regarding admission, in utero transport, and administration of antenatal fetal therapies such as corticosteroids and magnesium sulphate (see section titled Therapies to Delay Birth/Improve Neonatal Outcome). Urine dipstick of a midstream specimen (and culture in the laboratory if positive) will allow treatment of urinary tract infection if present.

If labour is considered established or imminent at a viable gestation, ultrasound (which can be performed at the bedside) is advised to determine fetal presentation, as well as liquor volume and placental site, if no previous scans are available. At the extremes of viability, performing an ultrasound EFW may provide prognostic information before delivery, and inform decisions about antenatal therapy to improve fetal outcome, and resuscitation decisions. Discussions involving the woman and her partner, and the obstetrician, midwife, and neonatologist regarding treatment and risks, mode of delivery, resuscitation, and likely course of treatment and outcome should be held before birth whenever possible, particularly in cases of extreme prematurity. Such discussions should include the prognosis for the infant (particularly important if the labour is extremely preterm), and the risks and benefits of interventions in labour and immediately postpartum, such as fetal monitoring and caesarean section. Consideration must also be given to the appropriate place of birth. If the appropriate level of neonatal care is not available in the obstetric unit, in utero transfer to a hospital with higher-level facilities should be carried out if it is considered safe to do so. If delivery is thought to be imminent, with risk of delivery en route to the facility, neonatal transfer should take place after birth once the infant is stabilised.

In cases of PPROM (particularly <34 weeks), routine care usually consists of hospital admission with regular monitoring of both maternal and fetal condition. Indications for delivery of the baby (by induction of labour or caesarean section depending on urgency, gestation, fetal status, presenting part, and maternal wishes) include concern about fetal condition (abnormal cardiotocography (CTG) or ultrasound assessment of well-being) and/or evidence of chorioamnionitis (raised serum inflammatory markers, maternal pyrexia, maternal or fetal tachycardia, or abdominal pain), as chorioamnionitis itself is a risk factor for an adverse neonatal outcome in PPROM,[99] as well as poor maternal outcome due to sepsis. It is worth noting that maternal fever is often a late sign in clinical chorioamnionitis. Although widely used, the clinical utility of serum inflammatory markers such as C-reactive protein have a poor correlation with histological chorioamnionitis[100,101] and fetal outcome. On hospital admission, an ultrasound examination is preferably performed to determine or confirm the gestational age, the presenting part of the fetus, the risk of umbilical cord prolapse (especially in case of a non-descended vertex or nonvertex presentation), the EFW, and the amniotic fluid compartment by means of either a single deepest pocket or an Amniotic Fluid Index (AFI) measurement.

Specific management options for PPROM are determined by gestational age, with the related risks of intrauterine infection and prematurity. There are two treatment approaches: 1) expectant management with surveillance of maternal and fetal condition; and 2) delivery by either induction of labour or caesarean section. Mid-trimester PPROM is associated with high perinatal mortality and morbidity[102] with a risk of the development of pulmonary hypoplasia secondary to oligohydramnios, together with the risks of prematurity itself. Thus, prior to neonatal viability, management options are limited, and a 'wait-and-see' policy is advised. Hospital admission is deferred until viability is reached, which means 24 weeks' gestation in most developed countries and after shared decision-making together with the parents. Because of high morbidity and mortality rates, a termination of pregnancy should be discussed as a potential option. If an expectant management approach is adopted, the pregnant woman is instructed to report to the hospital in case of a rise in temperature, foul-smelling purulent discharge, abdominal pain or contractions, blood loss, or signs of a prolapsed cord. Temperature can be monitored at home twice per day. Regular check-ups to monitor growth and amniotic fluid compartment at least every two weeks are advised, until 24 weeks.

After viability (defined in most units as 24 weeks' gestation, though discussions regarding viability must be made with the multi-disciplinary team and the woman herself) and after counselling on when to start active management with the obstetrician and neonatologist (prematurity is generally considered the greater risk vs those associated with PPROM), expectant management is usually undertaken. Patients may be managed as inpatients or outpatients, with regular attention paid to signs of intra-amniotic infection, placental abruption, cord prolapse, or progressive spontaneous PTL.[103]

Worldwide, no consensus has been reached so far regarding the best treatment in case of PPROM at 34–36[+6] weeks' gestation, and considerable variation in guidelines exist (see the Online Appendix). In 2010, Buchanan *et al.* reviewed the available evidence on the effect of planned early birth versus expectant management for women with PPROM <37 weeks' gestation.[104] They found that planned early birth was not associated with improved perinatal survival or reduced perinatal morbidity but there was a reduction in the incidence of chorioamnionitis if delivery was within 24 hours of presentation. For the mother, the authors found that early delivery may be associated with an increase in caesarean section rate. In 2012, the PPROMEXIL trial showed a low risk of neonatal sepsis (4.1% in the case of expectant management) after PPROM, with no reduction of this risk after induction of labour (2.6%; RR: 0.64; 95% CI: 0.25–1.6).[105,106] This was echoed by a trial by Morris *et al.* in which infants randomised to the immediate delivery group had increased rates of respiratory distress, requirement for ventilation and intensive care compared with those managed expectantly.[107] There may, however, be disadvantages with conservative management beyond 34[+0] weeks' gestation in the presence of known GBS colonisation, and in this group, early intervention may be preferable.[108] The 2017 Cochrane meta-analysis exploring the effect of planned delivery versus expectant management for women with PPROM concluded that expectant management with careful monitoring was safe, and in pregnancies over 34 weeks' gestation, associated with improved fetal and maternal outcomes versus planned delivery.[109] It is worth noting that evidence for expectant management has largely been extrapolated from trials of PPROM in infants between 34 and 37 weeks' gestation. Randomised controlled trials of management of PPROM at lower gestational ages have not been performed, and while the risks of prematurity increase at lower gestational ages, so may the impact of chorioamnionitis on the expectantly managed very premature fetus with PPROM.

Rupture of the fetal membranes at term (>37 weeks) before onset of labour is a frequently encountered obstetrical problem, occurring in 8–10% of cases. More than 60% of women will start delivering within 24 hours, when a policy of waiting for spontaneous labour is adopted. Fewer than 5% will not have started delivering within 72 hours after PROM.[110] In a Cochrane review, no differences were detected between planned delivery (within 24 hours of PROM) and expectant groups regarding the risk of caesarean section or operative vaginal birth, but lower rates of maternal infection (chorioamnionitis and endometritis) were observed in the planned delivery group.[111] Thus, in most national guidelines, it is recommended to offer induction of labour after PROM at term within 24–48 hours after rupture of membranes.

Therapies to Delay Birth/Improve Neonatal Outcome

Tocolysis

Although it has not been shown to improve neonatal outcomes, the use of tocolytic therapy – in order to delay delivery and allow in utero transfer or administration of antenatal corticosteroids and magnesium sulphate for neuroprotection – is common obstetric practice between 24 and 34 weeks' gestation. Many different drugs have been evaluated as tocolytic therapy: β-sympathomimetics (e.g. ritodrine and terbutaline),[112] calcium channel blockers (e.g. nifedipine),[113] prostaglandin inhibitors (e.g. indomethacin),[114] and oxytocin receptor blockers (e.g. atosiban)[115] are the most commonly used, each with a unique mode of action and side-effect profile. Each of these medications has been shown to reduce the incidence of delivery within 48 hours and up to seven days compared with placebo, but with no observed associated improvement in neonatal outcome. Owing to the higher incidence of maternal side effects associated with use of β-sympathomimetics (e.g. chest pain, tachycardia, palpitations, tremor, headaches, hyperglycaemia, hypokalaemia, nausea, and vomiting),[112] calcium channel blockers, prostaglandin inhibitors, and oxytocin receptor blockers are the most commonly used, though their use is often unlicensed (e.g. nifedipine, ritodrine), whereas atosiban is licensed in Europe (but not the USA) for use as a tocolytic. An individual participant data meta-analysis[116] comparing atosiban and nifedipine demonstrated comparable prolongation of pregnancy, but there was a small non-statistically significant increase in neonatal mortality (R: 1.4; 95% CI: 0.6–3.4) in the nifedipine group. As a result, some practitioners have a preference for the use of the more expensive atosiban as the tocolytic of choice.

After 48 hours of use, maintenance therapy with tocolytics is not beneficial[117,118] and may be associated with harm.[119] In general, the use of tocolytics after PPROM is not advised due to concern about risk of chorioamniontitis;[120] however, evidence informing this recommendation is based on small low-quality trials of drugs, many of which are no longer in use, and randomised trials are ongoing in this area.

Antenatal Corticosteroids

The administration of antenatal corticosteroids to women at high risk of PTB has been shown to enhance fetal lung maturity and confer morbidity and mortality advantages to the neonate, and has been an established treatment for women at high risk of preterm delivery for the last 30 years. Discovered incidentally by Liggins in 1969 while researching the impact of dexamethasone on preterm parturition in a sheep model, an RCT followed in 1972 ($n = 282$) in women with PTL at <37 weeks' gestation using betamethasone for the prevention of RDS.[121] A reduction of 11% in neonatal death and 20% in RDS was observed in the treatment group when compared with placebo. After a flurry of clinical trials in this area, the first meta-analysis was published by Crowley *et al.*, including 12 studies and over 3,000 women, which demonstrated that a course of antenatal corticosteroids reduced RDS and neonatal mortality by approximately 50% in infants born <34 weeks' gestation.[122] This has been confirmed by a 2020 Cochrane review that found an overall reduction in fetal and neonatal death, a reduction in RDS, and probably a reduction in interventricular haemorrhage and developmental delay at three years.[123] It is worth noting that many of these studies were performed prior to widespread use of surfactant for prevention and treatment of neonatal RDS, and so the benefit of antenatal corticosteroids may not be as pronounced in settings of modern neonatal care.

The timing of steroid administration is crucial to conferring benefit.[124] In the original meta-analysis, steroid-associated reduction in fetal and neonatal death is only seen in infants born within 24 and 48 hours, but not in those born between one and seven days or after seven days. The reduction in RDS was observed between 24 hours and seven days after administration, but not after seven.[125] This is particularly important, given that the majority of women who present with preterm contractions do not deliver within seven days but may still deliver preterm; thus, many receive steroids but deliver only after the benefit has been lost.

While conferring tremendous health benefit to the premature infant if given appropriately, the use of steroids is not without risk. There may be a small reduction in birthweight in infants treated with steroids, particularly those born more than seven days after administration, though the 2020 Cochrane analysis suggests little or no effect on birthweight.[123] There are, however, increasing concerns that fetal exposure to antenatal corticosteroids might be associated with physical, mental, and developmental disorders later in life.[126,127] Given that a large proportion of infants exposed to antenatal corticosteroids are subsequently born at term, accurate prediction of those at highest risk of PTB is therefore vital.[128]

Concerns regarding ubiquitous and liberal steroid use in women with threatened PTL were further raised after the WHO multi-country cluster RCT of corticosteroid use in low- and middle-income countries revealed increased risk of neonatal mortality in newborns who received antenatal corticosteroids, particularly in those infants who were subsequently born at or close to term, as well as an increased odds ratio for suspected maternal infection amongst those who received steroids.[129] That the majority of women who received steroids did not give birth to an infant <5th centile (a proxy measure for gestational prematurity) highlighted the need for caution regarding the over-diagnosis of suspected PTL and liberal use of steroids in infants who later deliver close to term, as well as concern regarding worsening infectious maternal and potentially fetal morbidity in infants who receive steroids.

. The effect of repetitive courses of corticosteroids in cases of PTL have been summarised in a Cochrane review of a total of more than 2,000 women.[130] Repeated courses were associated with a reduction in RDS and a reduction in composite serious infant outcomes, at the expense of a slight reduction in mean birthweight (mean difference: −75.79 g). However, due to the concerns regarding the fetal effects of repeated courses of steroids, particularly on growth, and theoretical concerns regarding glucose homeostasis and brain development, particularly for infants born near to term, there is significant variation in practice, and the use of more than two courses is not advocated. It is the opinion of the authors that a 'rescue' single dose of antenatal corticosteroids should be considered in women <32 weeks' gestation, who have received a course of steroids more than one week previously, but in whom the risk of premature delivery within 48 hours remains high. More important, however, is accurately timing steroid administration so as to reduce the incidence of steroids being given too early, and reduce the need for repeat doses, and inappropriate administration to infants destined to deliver at term. It is likely that use of predictive biomarkers and tests can aid this decision, enabling clinicians to move away from the traditional paradigm of giving steroids early in all cases of threatened PTL without consideration of the spectrum of risk, and the optimal timing to confer benefit, and avoid the need for repeated courses and treatment of the eventual term infant if possible.

Magnesium Sulphate

Preterm-birth-related brain injury and the associated neurodevelopmental consequences are characterised by diffuse white matter injury and/or intraventricular and intraparenchymal haemorrhage, cystic periventricular leukomalacia, and neuronal injury and loss. It is thought that ascending intra-amniotic infection and the associated fetal inflammatory response syndrome triggers oxidative stress, microglial activation, and neuronal excitotoxicity, leading to glutamate toxicity, affecting, among others, the vulnerable oligodendroglial progenitor cells, most susceptible to injury between 24 and 34 weeks' gestation.[131,132] While the exact mechanisms are unknown, prenatal administration of magnesium sulphate in cases with extremely PTL (originally as a tocolytic although it is in fact ineffective in this role) has been shown to have neuroprotective effects.[133] It is thought to act by preventing post-hypoxic glutamate-mediated neurotoxicity through acting as a non-competitive antagonist of the *N*-methyl-D-aspartic acid (NMDA) receptor on oligodendroglial progenitor cells and blocking excess release of glutamate.[134]

Several meta-analyses and a Cochrane review have demonstrated that giving intrapartum magnesium sulphate reduces the incidence of cerebral palsy and substantial gross motor dysfunction when the baby is born preterm.[135,136] There is no international consensus regarding the optimal dose and timing; guidelines vary between institutions. The most common dosing regime is that used for pre-eclampsia: a 4 g bolus, followed by an infusion of 1 g/hour for 24 hours. It should only be given if preterm delivery is imminent (within the next 24 hours), but it is not yet clear whether a post-bolus infusion is necessary, or whether repeated bolus doses of magnesium sulphate should be given if delivery does not occur when initially expected. While the greatest benefit is seen in infants born <30 weeks' gestation, national guidelines vary, with consideration for use up to 34 weeks' gestation (Online Appendix); research is needed to establish potential benefit for infants born after 30 weeks' gestation.

Antibiotic Therapy

With the strong association between infection and PPROM, being either cause or consequence, research has focused on the use of antibiotics following PPROM for the purpose of preventing infectious complications for both mother and child. In the 2013 Cochrane review, 22 trials were included involving over 6,000 women and their babies.[137] Different types of antibiotic regimes were prescribed, consisting mainly of broad-spectrum penicillins alone or in combination, or macrolide antibiotics (erythromycin) alone or in combination. Short-term benefits of antibiotic use included fewer cases of chorioamnionitis, babies born within 48 hours and within seven days after randomisation, neonatal infection, need for surfactant and oxygen therapy, and abnormal cerebral ultrasound before discharge from the hospital. Co-amoxiclav, however, was associated with an increased risk of neonatal NEC (RR: 4.72; 95% CI: 1.57–14.23). Most guidelines advocate use of erythromycin for 10 days for women with PPROM, though evidence of long-term neonatal benefit is lacking.[138]

In women with threatened PTL and intact membranes, use of antibiotics is not recommended and may be harmful. The ORACLE II multicenter trial[139] randomised over 6,000 women in threatened spontaneous PTL with intact membranes and no clinical evidence of infection. They received various combinations of penicillin and erythromycin regimes four times daily for 10 days or until delivery. None of the antibiotic combinations was associated with neonatal benefit, and a statistically non-significant increase in NEC was observed in the infants of women prescribed co-amoxiclav, mirroring the effect seen in women with PPROM. Furthermore, a seven-year follow-up of 3,196 infants involved in the ORACLE II trial revealed that the prescription of erythromycin ($\pm$ co-amoxiclav) was associated with functional impairment and an increased incidence of cerebral palsy.[140] Therefore, routine antibiotic treatment for prevention of PTL is not recommended. However, for women colonised with vaginal GBS, the leading cause of serious neonatal sepsis in developed countries, intrapartum intravenous penicillin started early in labour will prevent the majority (approximately 75%) of early onset infections.[141]

Labour and Delivery

Once premature delivery is thought to be inevitable, delivery must be attended by the obstetric and neonatal teams. If the delivery is taking place in a unit without appropriate neonatal facilities appropriate to the gestational age of the infant, and the window of opportunity for an in utero transfer has been lost, arrangements must be made to transfer the neonate once stabilised to a more appropriate care setting. Mode of delivery must be considered and discussed with the woman and her partner. Unfortunately, the optimal mode of delivery of the preterm infant has remained a controversial topic, with a lack of robust RCTs to provide evidence to guide these decisions; as a result, studies have yielded conflicting results. The largest study, published in 2012, is a non-randomised study comparing the mode of delivery of 2,885 singleton, preterm, small-for-gestational-age infants born with vertex presentation between 25 and 34 weeks' gestation.[142] No significant differences between neonatal death or contributors to neonatal morbidity (intraventricular and subdural haemorrhage, seizure or sepsis) were seen between the groups, though infants born by caesarean section had an increased incidence of RDS and a 5-minute Apgar score of <7 compared with those delivered vaginally. However, this study was non-randomised and therefore carries an inherent risk of bias associated with clinician 'choice'. For example, caesarean section may have been performed in patients who needed more urgent delivery (e.g. fetal compromise), thereby potentially leading to a more favourable outcome with vaginal delivery.

A Cochrane review of randomised studies comparing planned caesarean section with planned vaginal delivery concluded that there is not yet enough reliable evidence to compare planned caesarean delivery with planned vaginal delivery, as all four trials were stopped early owing to the inherent difficulties in recruiting women.[143] Therefore, decisions regarding mode of delivery remain based on hospital practice and clinician and patient preference. However, consideration must be given to the risks associated with caesarean section, including sepsis, maternal haemorrhage, and implications for future pregnancies such as the need for repeat caesarean section, uterine rupture, and placenta accreta. Before 26 weeks' gestation, the lower uterine segment has not yet fully formed, and a classical or De Lee (vertical) incision may be required for delivery of the baby, with increased risk of scar dehiscence in a subsequent pregnancy, compared with a lower transverse incision. In practice, as a result of difficulties in diagnosing PTL, a policy of caesarean section over vaginal delivery for preterm infants may lead to the delivery of infants earlier than they otherwise would have been born 'naturally', as waiting for confirmation of advanced labour may mean that the window for caesarean section has been lost.

With breech presentation there is insufficient evidence concerning preterm age categories, and the decision needs to be based on hospital practice and clinician and patient opinion. However, there is a risk of cord prolapse and head entrapment during preterm delivery, as well as term delivery.[144] If assisted vaginal delivery is necessary in a PTB, vacuum extraction is not recommended <34 weeks' gestation because of the increased risk of cephalhematoma, intracranial haemorrhage, and neonatal jaundice compared to term infants.[145,146,147] There is insufficient evidence to establish safety in infants between 34 and 37 weeks' gestation. Finally, the risk of hypoxia and progressive acidemia is higher in preterm infants, and CTG interpretation is somewhat more difficult in infants <28 weeks' gestation. For infants at the extreme limits of viability, the decision to monitor the baby with CTG must be discussed with the parents, particularly if the decision has been made not to intervene if fetal compromise becomes apparent. In general, most clinicians manage PTL as term labour, with the goal of eventual vaginal delivery. Large, well-designed intention-to-treat RCTs are required to aid this decision-making.

For women with PPROM, particular attention should be given to signs of intrauterine infection and the appropriate commencement of antibiotic therapy when present or in cases with a positive GBS culture or PCR test. In a Cochrane review that included 11 studies (1,296 women), no definite decision could be made as to the best treatment strategy, in terms of choice of antibiotic, dosage, and duration.[148] Limited evidence is available on whether continuing antibiotics in the postpartum period is advisable.

Once the baby is delivered, there is strong evidence to suggest that delaying cord clamping confers benefit to the preterm newborn. A Cochrane review compared immediate with delayed cord clamping (ranging from 30 to 120 seconds) for infants born <37 weeks' gestation,[149] showing an associated reduction in need for blood transfusions, incidence of low blood pressure, and incidence of intraventricular haemorrhage in the delayed group. However, in the event of postpartum haemorrhage or placenta previa, or if the neonate is asphyxiated and requires immediate resuscitation, immediate cord clamping may be required, or mechanisms to resuscitate them placed near to the mother for instigation prior to cord clamping. Further trials are under way to evaluate the benefits of this practice.

Threatened and Actual PTL and PPROM

SUMMARY OF MANAGEMENT OPTIONS

Management Options

Pre-pregnancy (Previous PTB/Other Risk Factors)
- Discuss the risk of recurrence in future pregnancy in women with a previous PTB, mid-trimester loss, PPROM, or other risk factors.
- Discuss management options for a future pregnancy.
- Advise about smoking, alcohol, recreational drugs, and weight.

Prenatal (See Online Appendix for Detailed Guideline Recommendations)

Screening (High-Risk Women)
- Vigilance for clinical features of recurrence
- Regular transvaginal cervical ultrasound examination
- fFN
- Other biochemical tests need further evaluation
- No evidence to support use of infection screening

Prophylaxis (High-Risk Women)
- Cervical cerclage is undertaken on the basis of the history and/or cervical ultrasound changes.
- 'Rescue cerclage' has limited evidence to support its use. It is best used in selected cases by experienced surgeons after careful counselling about risks and benefits.

(Cont.)

- Progesterone: vaginal pessary is of proven benefit. 17-OHP requires further evidence.
- Arabin pessary has limited data.

Diagnosis of PPROM

- Clinical (history and sterile speculum examination)
- pH and ferning tests have a risk of false-positive results
- IGFB-1 and PAMG-1 may be useful additional tests, although IGFB-1 has a risk of false-positive results
- Ultrasound examination of AFI is not helpful in equivocal cases
- Avoid digital vaginal examination unless the woman is in labour

Diagnosis of PTL (with Intact Membranes)

- Clinical assessment: gestational age, uterine activity, cervical dilatation, bleeding, fetal position and lie, vigilance for infection, search for cause or precipitating factor
- Transvaginal ultrasound assessment of CL if cervix not clinically dilated (useful in deciding management options)
- Biochemical screening:
  - fFN
  - phIGFBP-1 and PAMG-1 require further evaluation
- Formal risk assessment (e.g. QUiPP)

Presentation with Threatened or Actual PTL

- Initial assessment
  - Clinical assessment
  - Confirm gestational age
  - Estimate fetal weight with ultrasound and presentation
  - Multi-disciplinary discussion (i.e. including obstetrician neonatal paediatrician, and nursing and midwifery staff). Points covered would include plans for delivery (including place of birth), treatment options and mode of delivery
  - Involve woman and partner in all management discussions
- Treatments (see Online Appendix for detailed options)
  - Antenatal corticosteroids: recommended in all guidelines between 24^{+0} and 33^{+6} weeks; differences in recommendations for 22^{+0}–24^{+0}

(Cont.)

and 34^{+0}–36^{+6} weeks; consider repeating a single dose if undelivered >7 days

- Tocolysis: several drug choices; differences in guidelines regarding duration
- Magnesium sulphate: especially effective and recommended <30 weeks; guidelines vary in recommendations for 30^{+0}–34^{+6} weeks
- Antibiotics: up to 10 days treatment with erythromycin (+/- ampicillin) with PPROM; with PTL and intact membranes only consider using antibiotics in GBS carriers; do not use co-amoxiclav

Labour and Delivery

- Involve woman and partner in all management discussions.
- Place of delivery: this should take place where there are appropriate neonatal facilities but the transfer of a woman in PTL carries risks
- Obstetric, neonatal, nursing, and midwifery teams should be in place.
- Mode of delivery: optimum mode of delivery is not clear (see recommendations in the Online Appendix)
- Timing of delivery with PPROM (see recommendations in the Online Appendix)
- Other delivery issues:
  - Caesarean section with increasing prematurity has risks, especially <26 weeks (poorly developed lower segment).
  - Vaginal delivery of preterm breech presentation has risk of cord prolapse.
  - Vacuum delivery should be avoided <34 weeks.
  - Interpretation of fetal heart rate recording needs to take account of gestational age.
  - Vigilance for infection should be maintained with PPROM.
  - Deferring cord clamping by up to two minutes is of benefit (in the absence of major postpartum haemorrhage or placenta previa or fetal compromise).

Further Reading

Asztalos, EV, Murphy, KE, Matthews, SG. A growing dilemma: antenatal corticosteroids and long-term consequence. Am J Perinatol 2022; 39: 592–600.

Blencowe, H, Cousens, S, Chou, D, *et al*. Born too soon: the global epidemiology of 15 million preterm births. Reprod Health 2013; 10 (Suppl. 1): S2.

Carter, J, Seed, PT, Watson, HA, *et al*. Development and validation of prediction models for the QUiPP App v.2: a tool for predicting preterm birth in women with symptoms of threatened preterm labor. Ultrasound Obstet Gynecol 2019, 55(3): 357–67.

Evaluating Progestogens for Preventing Preterm Birth International Collaborative (EPPPIC): meta-analysis of individual participant data from randomised controlled trials. Lancet 2021; 397(10280): 1183–94.

Goldenberg, RL, Culhane, JF, Iams, JD, Romero, R. Epidemiology and causes of preterm birth. Lancet 2008; 371: 75–84.

Romero, R, Mazor, M, Munoz, H, *et al*. The preterm labor syndrome. Ann N Y Acad Sci 1994; 734: 414–29.

Shennan, AH, Story, L; the Royal College of Obstetricians, Gynaecologists. Cervical cerclage. BJOG 2022; 129: 1178–210.

References

1. World Health Organization. WHO: recommended definitions, terminology and format for statistical tables related to the perinatal period and use of a new certificate for cause of perinatal deaths. Modifications recommended by FIGO as amended October 14, 1976. Acta Obstet Gynecol Scand 1977; 56: 247–53.

2. Goldenberg, RL, Culhane, JF, Iams, JD, Romero, R. Epidemiology and causes of preterm birth. Lancet 2008; 371: 75–84.

3. Cox, SM, Williams, ML, Leveno, KJ. The natural history of preterm ruptured membranes: what to expect of expectant management. Obstet Gynecol 1988; 71: 558–62.

4. Steer, P. The epidemiology of preterm labor. BJOG 2005; 112 (Suppl. 1): 1–3.

5. Bates, E, Rouse, DJ, Mann, ML, et al. Neonatal outcomes after demonstrated fetal lung maturity before 39 weeks of gestation. Obstet Gynecol 2010; 116: 1288–95.

6. Blencowe, H, Cousens, S, Chou, D, et al. Born too soon: the global epidemiology of 15 million preterm births. Reprod Health 2013; 10 (Suppl. 1): S2.

7. Marlow, N. Full term: an artificial concept. Arch Dis Child Fetal Neonatal Ed 2012; 97: F158–9.

8. Blencowe, H, Cousens, S, Oestergaard, MZ, et al. National, regional, and worldwide estimates of preterm birth rates in the year 2010 with time trends since 1990 for selected countries: a systematic analysis and implications. Lancet 2012; 379: 2162–72.

9. Lawn, J, Kerber, K, Enweronu-Laryea, C, Cousens, S. 3.6 million neonatal deaths: what is progressing and what is not? Semin Perinatol 2010; 34: 371–86.

10. Chawanpaiboon, S, Vogel, JP, Moller, AB, et al. Global, regional, and national estimates of levels of preterm birth in 2014: a systematic review and modelling analysis. Lancet Glob Health 2019; 7(1): e37–46.

11. Naeye, RL, Ross, SM. Amniotic fluid infection syndrome. Clin Obstet Gynecol 1982; 9: 593–607.

12. Goncalves, LF, Chaiworapongsa, T, Romero, R. Intrauterine infection and prematurity. Ment Retard Dev Disabil Res Rev 2002; 8: 3–13.

13. Romero, R, Mazor, M, Munoz, H, et al. The preterm labor syndrome. Ann N Y Acad Sci 1994; 734: 414–29.

14. Romero, R, Dey, SK, Fisher, SJ. Preterm labor: one syndrome, many causes. Science 2014; 345: 760–5.

15. Winkvist, A, Mogren, I, Högberg, U. Familial patterns in birth characteristics: impact on individual and population risks. Int J Epidemiol 1998; 27: 248–54.

16. Shah, PS, Shah, V. Influence of the maternal birth status on offspring: a systematic review and meta-analysis. Acta Obstet Gynecol Scand 2009; 88: 1307–18. http://dx.doi.org/10.3109/00016340903358820.

17. Strauss, JF, Romero, R, Gomez-Lopez, N, *et al*. Spontaneous preterm birth: advances toward the discovery of genetic predisposition. Am J Obstet Gynecol 2018; 218: 294–314.e2. http://dx.doi.org/10.1016/j.ajog.2017 .12.009.

18. Esplin, MS, Manuck, TA, Varner, MW, *et al*. Cluster analysis of spontaneous preterm birth phenotypes identifies potential associations among preterm birth mechanisms. Am J Obstet Gynecol 2015; 213: 429.e1–9. http://dx.doi.org/10.1016/j.ajog.2015.06.011.

19. Menon, R, Velez, DR, Thorsen, P, *et al*. Ethnic differences in key candidate genes for spontaneous preterm birth: TNF-alpha and its receptors. Hum Hered 2006; 62: 107–18.

20. Moore, T, Hennessy, EM, Myles, J, *et al*. Neurological and developmental outcome in extremely preterm children born in England in 1995 and 2006: the EPICure studies. BMJ 2012; 345: e7961.

21. Wood, N, Costeloe, K, Gibson, A, *et al*. The EPICure study: associations and antecedents of neurological and developmental disability at 30 months of age following extremely preterm birth. Arch Dis Child Fetal Neonatal Ed 2005; 90: F134–40.

22. Mangham, LJ, Petrou, S, Doyle, LW, Draper, ES, Marlow, N. The cost of preterm birth throughout childhood in England and Wales. Pediatrics 2009; 123: e312–27.

23. Butler, AS, Behrman, RE. Preterm Birth: Causes, Consequences, and Prevention. Washington, DC: National Academies Press, 2007.

24. Goldenberg, RL, Iams, JD, Mercer, BM, *et al*. The preterm prediction study: the value of new vs standard risk factors in predicting early and all spontaneous preterm births. NICHD MFMU Network. Am J Public Health 1998; 88: 233–8.

25. Mercer, BM, Goldenberg, RL, Moawad, AH, *et al*. The preterm prediction study: effect of gestational age and cause of preterm birth on subsequent obstetric outcome. Am J Obstet Gynecol 1999; 181: 1216–21.

26. McManemy, J, Cooke, E, Amon, E, Leet, T. Recurrence risk for preterm delivery. Am J Obstet Gynecol 2007; 196: 576.e1–6.

27. Crane, JM, Delaney, T, Hutchens, D. Transvaginal ultrasonography in the prediction of preterm birth after treatment for cervical intraepithelial neoplasia. Obstet Gynecol 2006; 107: 37–44.

28. Levine, LD, Sammel, MD, Hirshberg, A, Elovitz, MA, Srinivas, SK. Does stage of labor at time of cesarean delivery affect risk of subsequent preterm birth? Am J Obstet Gynecol 2015; 212: 360.e1–7. http://dx.doi.org/10.1016/j.ajog.2014.09.035.

29. Watson, HA, Ridout, A, Shennan, AH. Second stage cesarean as risk factor for preterm birth: how to manage subsequent pregnancies? Am J Obstet Gynecol 2018; 218: 367–8. http://dx.doi.org/10.1016/j.ajog.2017.11.589.

30. Van Winsen, KD, Savvidou, MD, Steer, PJ. The effect of mode of delivery and duration of labor on subsequent pregnancy outcomes: a retrospective cohort study. BJOG 2021; 128(13): 2132–9. http://dx.doi.org/10.1111/1471-0528.16864.

31. Homer, HA, Li, TC, Cooke, ID. The septate uterus: a review of management and reproductive outcome. Fertil Steril 2000; 73: 1–14.

32. Brett, K, Strogatz, D, Savitz, D. Employment, job strain, and preterm delivery among women in North Carolina. Am J Public Health 1997; 87: 199–204.

33. Smith, LK, Draper, ES, Manktelow, BN, Doring, JS, Field, JA. Socioeconomic inequalities in very preterm birth rates. Arch Dis Child Fetal Neonatal Ed 2007; 92: F11–14.

34. Menon, R, Fortunato, SJ, Edwards, DR, Williams, SM. Association of genetic variants, ethnicity and preterm birth with amniotic fluid cytokine concentrations. Ann Hum Genet 2010; 74: 165–83.

35. Heath, V, Southall, T, Souka, A, Novakov, A, Nikolaides, KH. Cervical length at 23 weeks of gestation: relation to demographic characteristics and previous obstetric history. Ultrasound Obst Gynecol 1998; 12: 304–11.

36. Iams, JD, Goldenberg, RL, Meis, PJ, *et al.* The length of the cervix and the risk of spontaneous premature delivery. N Eng J Med 1996; 334: 567–73.

37. To, M, Skentou, C, Chan, C, Zagaliki, A, Nikolaides, KH. Cervical assessment at the routine 23-week scan: standardizing techniques. Ultrasound Obst Gynecol 2001; 17: 217–19.

38. Guzman, E, Walters, C, Ananth, C, *et al.* A comparison of sonographic cervical parameters in predicting spontaneous preterm birth in high-risk singleton gestations. Ultrasound Obst Gynecol 2001; 18: 204–10.

39. Owen, J, Yost, N, Berghella, V, *et al.* Midtrimester endovaginal sonography in women at high risk for spontaneous preterm birth. JAMA 2001; 286: 1340–8.

40. Cook, CM, Ellwood, D. The cervix as a predictor of preterm delivery in 'at-risk' women. Ultrasound Obst Gynecol 2000; 15: 109–13.
41. Lim, AC, Hegeman, MA, Huis In 'T Veld, MA, *et al*. Cervical length measurement for the prediction of preterm birth in multiple pregnancies: a systematic review and bivariate meta-analysis. Ultrasound Obst Gynecol 2011; 38: 10–17.
42. Goepfert, AR, Goldenberg, RL, Mercer, B, *et al*. The Preterm Prediction Study: quantitative fetal fibronectin values and the prediction of spontaneous preterm birth. Am J Obstet Gynecol 2000; 183: 1480–3.
43. Abbott, DA, Hezelgrave, NL, Seed, PT, *et al*. Quantitative fetal fibronectin to predict preterm birth in asymptomatic women at high risk. Obstet Gynecol 2015; 125: 1168–76.
44. Abbott, DS, Radford, SK, Seed, PT, Tribe, RM, Shennan, AH. Evaluation of a quantitative fetal fibronectin test for spontaneous preterm birth in symptomatic women. Am J Obstet Gynecol 2013; 208: 122.e1–6.
45. Amsel, R, Totten, PA, Spiegel, CA, *et al*. Nonspecific vaginitis: diagnostic criteria and microbial and epidemiologic associations. Am J Med 1983; 74: 14–22.
46. Leitich, H, Kiss, H. Asymptomatic bacterial vaginosis and intermediate flora as risk factors for adverse pregnancy outcome. Best Pract Res Clin Obstet Gynaecol 2007; 21: 375–90.
47. Brocklehurst, P, Gordon, A, Heatley, E, Milan, SJ. Antibiotics for treating bacterial vaginosis in pregnancy. Cochrane Database Syst Rev 2013; (1): CD000262.
48. Vermeulen, GM, Bruinse, HW. Prophylactic administration of clindamycin 2% vaginal cream to reduce the incidence of spontaneous preterm birth in women with an increased recurrence risk: a randomised placebo-controlled double-blind trial. Br J Obstet Gynaecol 1999; 106: 652–7.
49. Shennan, A, Crawshaw, S, Briley, A, *et al*. A randomised controlled trial of metronidazole for the prevention of preterm birth in women positive for cervicovaginal fetal fibronectin: the PREMET Study. BJOG 2006; 113: 65–74.
50. Kurkinen-Räty, M, Vuopala, S, Koskela, M, *et al*. A randomised controlled trial of vaginal clindamycin for early pregnancy bacterial vaginosis. BJOG 2000; 107: 1427–32.
51. Nicolle, LE, Bradley, S, Colgan, R, *et al*. Infectious Diseases Society of America guidelines for the diagnosis and treatment of asymptomatic bacteriuria in adults. Clin Infect Dis 2005; 40: 643–54.

52. Villar, J, Gulmezoglu, AM, De Onis, M. Nutritional and antimicrobial interventions to prevent preterm birth: an overview of randomized controlled trials. Obstet Gynecol Surv 1998; 53: 575–85.

53. Smaill, FM, Vazquez, JC. Antibiotics for asymptomatic bacteriuria in pregnancy. Cochrane Database Syst Rev 2007; (8): CD000490.

54. Bianchi-Jassir, F, Seale, AC, Kohli-Lynch, M, *et al.* Preterm birth associated with Group B streptococcus maternal colonization worldwide: systematic review and meta-analyses. Clin Infect Dis 2017; 65(Suppl. 2): S133–42.

55. Macnaughton, M, Chalmers, I, Dubowitz, V, *et al.* Final report of the Medical Research Council/Royal College of Obstetricians and Gynaecologists multicentre randomised trial of cervical cerclage. Br J Obstet Gynaecol 1993; 100: 516–23.

56. Shennan, AH, Story, L. The Royal College of Obstetricians, Gynaecologists. Cervical cerclage. BJOG 2022; 129: 1178–210.

57. American College of Obstetricians and Gynecologists' Committee on Practice Bulletins – Obstetrics. Practice bulletin no. 142: cerclage for the management of cervical insufficiency. Obstet Gynecol 2014; 123: 372–9. http://dx.doi.org/10.1097/01.AOG.0000443276.68274.cc.

58. To, MS, Alfirevic, Z, Heath, VC, *et al.* Cervical cerclage for prevention of preterm delivery in women with short cervix: randomised controlled trial. Lancet 2004; 363: 1849–53.

59. Berghella, V, Odibo, AO, To, MS, Rust, OA, Althusius, SM. Cerclage for short cervix on ultrasonography: meta-analysis of trials using individual patient-level data. Obstet Gynecol 2005; 106: 181–9.

60. Althuisius, SM, Dekker, GA, Hummel, P, van Geijn, HP. Cervical incompetence prevention randomized cerclage trial: emergency cerclage with bed rest versus bed rest alone. Am J Obstet Gynecol 2003; 189: 907–10.

61. Chandiramani, M, Shennan, AH. Premature cervical change and the use of cervical cerclage. Fetal Maternal Med Rev 2007; 18: 25–52.

62. Odibo, AO, Berghella, V, To, MS, *et al.* Shirodkar versus McDonald cerclage for the prevention of preterm birth in women with short cervical length. Am J Perinatol 2007; 24: 55–60.

63. Shennan, A, Chandiramani, M, Bennett, P, *et al.* MAVRIC: a multicentre randomised controlled trial of transabdominal versus transvaginal cervical cerclage. Am J Obstet Gynecol 2019; 222(3): 261.e1–9. http://dx.doi.org/10.1016/j.ajog.2019.09.040.

64. Hodgetts Morton, V, Toozs-Hobson, P, Moakes, CA, *et al.* Monofilament suture versus braided suture thread to improve pregnancy outcomes after

vaginal cervical cerclage (C-STICH): a pragmatic randomised, controlled, phase 3, superiority trial. Lancet 2022; 400(10361): 1426–36.

65. Evaluating Progestogens for Preventing Preterm birth International Collaborative (EPPPIC): meta-analysis of individual participant data from randomised controlled trials. Lancet 2021; 397(10280): 1183–94.

66. Blackwell, SC, Gyamfi-Bannerman, C, Biggio, JR, Jr, *et al.* 17-OHPC to Prevent Recurrent Preterm Birth in Singleton Gestations (PROLONG Study): a multicenter, international, randomized double-blind trial. Am J Perinatol 2020; 37(2): 127–36. http://dx.doi.org/10.1055/s-0039-3400227.

67. Meis, PJ, Klebanoff, M, Thom, E, *et al.* Prevention of recurrent preterm delivery by 17 alpha-hydroxyprogesterone caproate. N Engl J Med 2003; 348: 2379–85.

68. Keirse, MJ. Progesterone and preterm: seventy years of 'deja vu' or 'still to be seen'? Birth 2004; 31: 230–5.

69. Iams, JD, Newman, RB, Thom, EA, *et al.* Frequency of uterine contractions and the risk of spontaneous preterm delivery. N Eng J Med 2002; 346: 250–5.

70. Romero, R, Yeo, L, Chaemsaithong, P, Chaiworapongsa, T, Hassan, SS. Progesterone to prevent spontaneous preterm birth. Semin Fetal Neonatal Med 2014; 19: 15–26.

71. Hassan, SS, Romero, R, Vidyadhari, D, *et al.*; PREGNANT trial. Vaginal progesterone reduces the rate of preterm birth in women with a sonographic short cervix: a multicenter, randomized, double-blind, placebo-controlled trial. Ultrasound Obstet Gynecol 2011; 38: 18–31. http://dx.doi.org/10.1002/uog.9017.

72. Conde-Agudelo, A, Romero, R. Does vaginal progesterone prevent recurrent preterm birth in women with a singleton gestation and a history of spontaneous preterm birth? Evidence from a systematic review and meta-analysis. Am J Obstet Gynecol 2022; 227(3): 440–61.e2. http://dx.doi.org/10.1016/j.ajog.2022.04.023.

73. Rode, L, Klein, K, Nicolaides, K, Krampl-Bettelheim, E, Tabor, A. Prevention of preterm delivery in twin gestations (PREDICT): a multicenter, randomized, placebo-controlled trial on the effect of vaginal micronized progesterone. Ultrasound Obstet Gynecol 2011; 38: 272–80.

74. Norman, JE, Mackenzie, F, Owen, P, *et al.* Progesterone for the prevention of preterm birth in twin pregnancy (STOPPIT): a randomised, double-blind, placebo-controlled study and meta-analysis. Lancet 2009; 373: 2034–40.

75. Wood, S, Ross, S, Tang, S, *et al.* Vaginal progesterone to prevent preterm birth in multiple pregnancy: a randomized controlled trial. J Perinat Med 2012; 40: 593–9.

76. Serra, V, Perales, A, Meseguer, J, *et al.* Increased doses of vaginal progesterone for the prevention of preterm birth in twin pregnancies: a randomised controlled double-blind multicentre trial. BJOG 2013; 120: 50–7.

77. Conde-Agudelo, A, Romero, R, Hassan, SS, Yeo, L. Transvaginal sonographic cervical length for the prediction of spontaneous preterm birth in twin pregnancies: a systematic review and metaanalysis. Am J Obstet Gynecol 2010; 203: 128.e1–12.

78. Goya, M, Pratcorona, L, Merced, C, *et al.* Cervical pessary in pregnant women with a short cervix (PECEP): an open-label randomised controlled trial. Lancet 2012; 379: 1800–6.

79. Nicolaides, KH, Syngelaki, A, Poon, LC, *et al.* A randomized trial of a cervical pessary to prevent preterm singleton birth. N Engl J Med 2016; 374(11): 1044–52. http://dx.doi.org/10.1056/NEJMoa1511014.

80. Hui, SY, Chor, CM, Lau, TK, Lao, TT, Leung, TY. Cerclage pessary for preventing preterm birth in women with a singleton pregnancy and a short cervix at 20 to 24 weeks: a randomized controlled trial. Am J Perinatol 2013; 30: 283–8.

81. Jin, XH, Li, D, Huang, LL. Cervical pessary for prevention of preterm birth: a meta-analysis. Sci Rep 2017; 7:: 42560. http://dx.doi.org/10.1038/srep42560

82. Norman, JE, Norrie, J, MacLennan, G, *et al.* The Arabin pessary to prevent preterm birth in women with a twin pregnancy and a short cervix: the STOPPIT 2 RCT. Health Technol Assess 2021; 25(44): 1–66.

83. Watson, HA, Seed, PT, Carter, J, *et al.* Development and validation of the predictive models for the QUiPP App v.2: a tool for predicting preterm birth in high-risk asymptomatic women. Ultrasound Obstet Gynecol 2020; 55(3): 348–56. http://dx.doi.org/10.1002/uog.20401.

84. Carter, J, Seed, PT, Watson, HA, *et al.* Development and validation of prediction models for the QUiPP App v.2: a tool for predicting preterm birth in women with symptoms of threatened preterm labor. Ultrasound Obstet Gynecol 2020; 55(3): 357–67. http://dx.doi.org/10.1002/uog.20422.

85. Watson, H, Carlisle, N, Seed, PT, *et al.* Evaluating the use of the QUiPP app and its impact on the management of threatened preterm labor: a cluster randomised trial. PLoS Med 2021; 18(7): e1003689.

86. Akercan, F, Kazandi, M, Sendag, F, *et al.* Value of cervical phosphorylated insulin like growth factor binding protein-1 in the prediction of preterm labor. J Reprod Med 2004; 49: 368–72.

87. Cooper, S, Lange, I, Wood, S, *et al.* Diagnostic accuracy of rapid phIGFBP-I assay for predicting preterm labor in symptomatic patients. J Perinatol 2011; 32: 460–5.

88. Petrunin, D, Griaznova, IM, Petrunina, I, Tatarinov, IS. Immunochemical identification of organ specific human placental alpha-1-globulin and its concentration in amniotic fluid. Akush Ginekol (Mosk) 1977; 1: 62–4.

89. Nikolova, T, Bayev, O, Nikolova, N, di Renzo, G. Evaluation of a novel placental alpha microglobulin-1 (PAMG-1) test to predict spontaneous preterm delivery. J Perinat Med 2014; 42: 473–7.

90. Fuchs, I, Henrich, W, Osthues, K, Dudenhausen, JW. Sonographic cervical length in singleton pregnancies with intact membranes presenting with threatened preterm labor. Ultrasound Obst Gynecol 2004; 24: 554–7.

91. Lewis, DF, Major, CA, Towers, CV, *et al.* Effects of digital vaginal examinations on latency period in preterm premature rupture of membranes. Obstet Gynecol 1992; 80: 630–4.

92. Alexander, JM, Mercer, BM, Miodovnik, M, *et al.* The impact of digital cervical examination on expectantly managed preterm rupture of membranes. Am J Obstet Gynecol 2000; 183: 1003–7.

93. Friedman, ML, McElin, TW. Diagnosis of ruptured fetal membranes: clinical study and review of the literature. Am J Obstet Gynecol 1969; 104: 544–50.

94. van der Ham, DP, van Teeffelen, AS, Mol, BW. Prelabor rupture of membranes: overview of diagnostic methods. Curr Opin Obstet Gynecol 2012; 24: 408–12.

95. Abdelazim, IA, Makhlouf, HH. Placental alpha microglobulin-1 (AmniSure test) versus insulin-like growth factor binding protein-1 (Actim PROM test) for detection of premature rupture of fetal membranes. J Obstet Gynaecol Res 2013; 39: 1129–36.

96. Sosa, CG, Herrera, E, Restrepo, JC, Strauss, A, Alonso, J. Comparison of placental alpha microglobulin-1 in vaginal fluid with intra-amniotic injection of indigo carmine for the diagnosis of rupture of membranes. J Perinat Med 2014; 42: 611–16.

97. Lee, SM, Romero, R, Park, JW, *et al.* The clinical significance of a positive Amnisure test in women with preterm labor and intact membranes. J Matern Fetal Neonatal Med 2012; 25: 1690–8.

98. Palacio, M, Kühnert, M, Berger, R, Larios, CL, Marcellin, L. Meta-analysis of studies on biochemical marker tests for the diagnosis of premature rupture of membranes: comparison of performance indexes. BMC Pregnancy Childbirth 2014; 14: 183. http://dx.doi.org/10.1186/1471-2393-14-183.

99. Ramsey, PS, Lieman, JM, Brumfield, CG, Carlo, W. Chorioamnionitis increases neonatal morbidity in pregnancies complicated by preterm premature rupture of membranes. Am J Obstet Gynecol 2005; 192: 1162–6.

100. van de Laar, R, van der Ham, DP, Oei, SG, *et al.* Accuracy of C-reactive protein determination in predicting chorioamnionitis and neonatal infection in pregnant women with premature rupture of membranes: a systematic review. Eur J Obstet Gynecol Reprod Biol 2009; 147: 124–9.

101. Trochez-Martinez, RD, Smith, P, Lamont, RF. Use of C-reactive protein as a predictor of chorioamnionitis in preterm prelabor rupture of membranes: a systematic review. BJOG 2007; 114: 796–801.

102. Waters, TP, Mercer, BM. The management of preterm premature rupture of the membranes near the limit of fetal viability. Am J Obstet Gynecol 2009; 201: 230–40.

103. Lewis, DF, Robichaux, AG, Jaekle, RK, *et al.* Expectant management of preterm premature rupture of membranes and nonvertex presentation: what are the risks? Am J Obstet Gynecol 2007; 196: 566.e1–5.

104. Buchanan, SL, Crowther, CA, Levett, KM, Middleton, P, Morris, J. Planned early birth versus expectant management for women with preterm prelabor rupture of membranes prior to 37 weeks' gestation for improving pregnancy outcome. Cochrane Database Syst Rev 2010; (3): CD004735.

105. van der Ham, DP, Nijhuis, JG, Mol, BW, *et al.* Induction of labor versus expectant management in women with preterm prelabor rupture of membranes between 34 and 37 weeks (the PPROMEXIL-trial). BMC Pregnancy Childbirth 2007; 7: 11.

106. van der Ham, DP, van der Heyden, JL, Opmeer, BC, *et al.* Management of late-preterm premature rupture of membranes: the PPROMEXIL-2 trial. Am J Obstet Gynecol 2012; 207: 276.e1–10.

107. Morris, JM, Roberts, CL, Bowen, JR, *et al.* PPROMT Collaboration. Immediate delivery compared with expectant management after preterm pre-labour rupture of the membranes close to term (PPROMT trial): a randomised controlled trial. Lancet 2016; 387(10017): 444–52.

108. Tajik, P, van der Ham, DP, Zafarmand, MH, *et al.* Using vaginal Group B streptococcus colonisation in women with preterm premature rupture of membranes to guide the decision for immediate delivery: a secondary analysis of the PPROMEXIL trials. BJOG 2014; 121: 1263–72.

109. Bond, DM, Middleton, P, Levett, KM, *et al.* Planned early birth versus expectant management for women with preterm prelabor rupture of membranes prior to 37 weeks' gestation for improving pregnancy outcome. Cochrane Database Syst Rev 2017; 3(3): CD004735. http://dx.doi.org/10.1002/14651858.CD004735.pub4.

110. Hannah, ME, Ohlsson, A, Farine, D, *et al.* Induction of labor compared with expectant management for prelabor rupture of the membranes at term. TERMPROM Study Group. N Engl J Med 1996; 334: 1005–10.

111. Dare, MR, Middleton, P, Crowther, CA, Flenady, VJ, Varatharaju, B. Planned early birth versus expectant management (waiting) for prelabor rupture of membranes at term (37 weeks or more). Cochrane Database Syst Rev 2006; (1): CD005302.

112. Anotayanonth, S, Subhedar, NV, Neilson, JP, Harigopal, S. Betamimetics for inhibiting preterm labor. Cochrane Database Syst Rev 2004; (4): CD004352.

113. King, JF, Flenady, VJ, Papatsonis, DN, *et al.* Calcium channel blockers for inhibiting preterm labour. Cochrane Database Syst Rev 2003; (1): CD002255. http://dx.doi.org/10.1002/14651858.CD002255. Update in: Cochrane Database Syst Rev 2014; 6: CD002255.

114. King, JF, Flenady, V, Cole, S, Thornton, S. Cyclo-oxygenase (COX) inhibitors for treating preterm labor. Cochrane Database Syst Rev 2005; (2): CD001992.

115. Papatsonis, D, Flenady, V, Liley, H. Maintenance therapy with oxytocin antagonists for inhibiting preterm birth after threatened preterm labour. Cochrane Database Syst Rev 2013; 10: CD005938.

116. van Winden, TMS, Nijman, TAJ, Kleinrouweler, CE, *et al.* Tocolysis with nifedipine versus atosiban and perinatal outcome: an individual participant data meta-analysis. BMC Pregnancy Childbirth 2022; 22(1): 567. http://dx.doi.org/10.1186/s12884-022-04854-1.

117. Mackeen, AD, Seibel-Seamon, J, Muhammad, J, *et al.* Tocolytics for preterm premature rupture of membranes. Cochrane Database Syst Rev 2014; (2): CD007062.

118. Naik Gaunekar, N, Raman, P, Bain, E, *et al.* Maintenance therapy with calcium channel blockers for preventing preterm birth after threatened preterm labor. Cochrane Database Syst Rev 2013; (10): CD004071.

119. van Vliet, E, Seinen, L, Roos, C, *et al.* Maintenance tocolysis with nifedipine in threatened preterm labour: 2-year follow up of the offspring in the APOSTEL II trial. BJOG 2016; 123(7): 1107–14.

120. Thornton, JG. Maintenance tocolysis. BJOG 2005; 112: 118–21.

121. Liggins, G. Premature delivery of foetal lambs infused with glucocorticoids. J Endocrinol 1969; 45: 515–23.

122. Crowley, P, Chalmers, I, Keirse, MJ. The effects of corticosteroid administration before preterm delivery: an overview of the evidence from controlled trials. Br J Obstet Gynaecol 1990; 97: 11–25.

123. McGoldrick, E, Stewart, F, Parker, R, Dalziel, SR. Antenatal corticosteroids for accelerating fetal lung maturation for women at risk of preterm birth. Cochrane Database Syst Rev 2020; (12): CD004454. http://dx.doi.org/10.1002/14651858.CD004454.pub4.

124. Melamed, N, Shah, J, Soraisham, A, *et al*. Association between antenatal corticosteroid administration-to-birth interval and outcomes of preterm neonates. Obstet Gynecol 2015; 125: 1377–84.

125. Roberts, D, Dalziel, S. Antenatal corticosteroids for accelerating fetal lung maturation for women at risk of preterm birth. Cochrane Database Syst Rev 2006; (3): CD004454.

126. Melamed, N, Asztalos, E, Murphy, K, *et al*. Neurodevelopmental disorders among term infants exposed to antenatal corticosteroids during pregnancy: a population-based study. BMJ Open 2019; 9: e031197.

127. Asztalos, EV, Murphy, KE, Matthews, SG. A growing dilemma: antenatal corticosteroids and long-term consequence. Am J Perinatol 2022; 39: 592–600.

128. Räikkönen, K, Gissler, M, Kajantie, E. Associations between maternal antenatal corticosteroid treatment and mental and behavioral disorders in children. JAMA 2020; 323: 1924–33.

129. Klein, K, McClure, EM, Colaci, D, *et al*. The Antenatal Corticosteroids Trial (ACT): a secondary analysis to explore site differences in a multi-country trial. Reprod Health 2016; 13(1): 64.

130. Hamm, RF, Combs, CA, Aghajanian, P, Friedman, AM; Patient Safety and Quality Committee. Society for Maternal–Fetal Medicine special statement: quality metrics for optimal timing of antenatal corticosteroid administration. Am J Obstet Gynecol 2022; 226: B2–10.

131. Crowther, CA, McKinlay, CJ, Middleton, P, Harding, JE. Repeat doses of prenatal corticosteroids for women at risk of preterm birth for improving neonatal health outcomes. Cochrane Database Syst Rev 2011; (6): CD003935.

132. Back, SA, Han, BH, Luo, NL, *et al*. Selective vulnerability of late oligodendrocyte progenitors to hypoxia–ischemia. J Neurosci 2002; 22: 455–63.

133. Haynes, RL, Folkerth, RD, Keefe, RJ, *et al*. Nitrosative and oxidative injury to premyelinating oligodendrocytes in periventricular leukomalacia. J Neuropathol Exp Neurol 2003; 62: 441–50.

134. McDonald, JW, Silverstein, FS, Johnston, MV. Magnesium reduces N-methyl-D-aspartate (NMDA)-mediated brain injury in perinatal rats. Neurosci Lett 1990; 109: 234–8.

References

135. Burd, I, Breen, K, Friedman, A, Chai, J, Elovitz, MA. Magnesium sulfate reduces inflammation-associated brain injury in fetal mice. Am J Obstet Gynecol 2010; 202: 292.e1–9.

136. Crowther, CA, Hiller, JE, Doyle, LW, Haslam, RR. Effect of magnesium sulfate given for neuroprotection before preterm birth: a randomized controlled trial. JAMA 2003; 290: 2669–76.

137. Doyle, LW, Crowther, CA, Middleton, P, Marret, S, Rouse, D. Magnesium sulphate for women at risk of preterm birth for neuroprotection of the fetus. Cochrane Database Syst Rev 2009; (1): CD004661.

138. Kenyon, S, Boulvain, M, Neilson, J. Antibiotics for preterm rupture of membranes. Cochrane Database Syst Rev 2013; (12): CD001058.

139. Kenyon, SL, Taylor, DJ, Tarnow-Mordi, W; ORACLE Collaborative Group. Broad-spectrum antibiotics for spontaneous preterm labor: the ORACLE II randomised trial. Lancet 2001; 357: 989–94.

140. Kenyon, S, Pike, K, Jones, DR, *et al.* Childhood outcomes after prescription of antibiotics to pregnant women with preterm rupture of the membranes: 7-year follow-up of the ORACLE I trial. Lancet 2008; 372: 1310–18.

141. Boyer, KM, Gotoff, SP. Prevention of early-onset neonatal Group B streptococcal disease with selective intrapartum chemoprophylaxis. New Eng J Med 1986; 314: 1665–9.

142. Werner, EF, Savitz, DA, Janevic, TM, *et al.* Mode of delivery and neonatal outcomes in preterm, small-for-gestational-age newborns. Obstet Gynecol 2012; 120: 560–4.

143. Alfirevic, Z, Milan, SJ, Livio, S. Cesarean section versus vaginal delivery for preterm birth in singletons. Cochrane Database Syst Rev 2012; (6): CD000078.

144. Hannah, ME, Hannah, WJ, Hewson, SA, *et al.* Planned cesarean section versus planned vaginal birth for breech presentation at term: a randomised multicentre trial. Term Breech Trial Collaborative Group. Lancet 2000; 356: 1375–83.

145. Rosemann, G. Vacuum extraction of premature infants. S Afr J Obstet Gynaecol 1969; 7: 10–12.

146. Åberg, K, Norman, M, Ekéus, C. Preterm birth by vacuum extraction and neonatal outcome: a population-based cohort study. BMC Pregnancy Childbirth 2014; 14: 42.

147. Royal College of Obstetricians and Gynaecologists. Operative Vaginal Delivery. Green-top Guideline No. 26. London: Royal College of Obstetricians and Gynaecologists, 2011. www.rcog.org.uk/en/guide lines-research-services/guidelines/gtg26/.

148. Chapman, E, Reveiz, L, Illanes, E, Bonfill Cosp, X. Antibiotic regimens for management of intra-amniotic infection. Cochrane Database Syst Rev 2014; (12): CD010976.

149. Rabe, H, Reynolds, G, Diaz-Rossello, J. Early versus delayed umbilical cord clamping in preterm infants. Cochrane Database Syst Rev 2004; (4): CD003248.

Cambridge Elements ☰

High-Risk Pregnancy: Management Options

Professor David James

Emeritus Professor, University of Nottingham, UK

David James was Professor of Fetomaternal Medicine at the University of Nottingham from 1992–2009. The post involved clinical service, especially the management of high-risk pregnancies, guideline development, research and teaching and NHS management. From 2009–14 he was Clinical Director of Women's Health at the National Centre for Clinical Excellence for Women's and Children's Health. He was also Clinical Lead for the RCOG/RCM/eLfH eFM E-Learning Project. He is a recognised authority on the management of problem/complicated pregnancies with over 200 peer-reviewed publications. He has published 16 books, the best-known being *High-Risk Pregnancy: Management Options*.

Professor Philip Steer

Emeritus Professor, Imperial College, London, UK

Philip Steer is Emeritus Professor of Obstetrics at Imperial College London, having been appointed Professor in 1989. He was a consultant obstetrician for 35 years. He was Editor-in-Chief of *BJOG – An International Journal of Obstetrics and Gynaecology* – from 2005–2012, and is now Editor Emeritus. He has published more than 150 peer-reviewed research papers, 109 reviews and editorials and 66 book chapters/books, the best known and most successful being *High-Risk Pregnancy: Management Options*. The fifth edition was published in 2018. He has been President of the British Association of Perinatal Medicine and President of the Section of Obstetrics and Gynaecology of the Royal Society of Medicine. He is an honorary fellow of the College of Obstetricians and Gynaecologists of South Africa, and of the American Gynecological & Obstetrical Society.

Professor Carl Weiner

Creighton University School of Medicine, Phoenix, AZ, USA

Carl Weiner is presently Head of Maternal Fetal Medicine for the CommonSpirit Health System, Arizona, Director of Maternal Fetal Medicine, Dignity St Joseph's Hospital, Professor, Obstetrics and Gynecology, Creighton School of Medicine, Phoenix, and Professor, College of Health Solutions, Arizona State University. He is the former Krantz Professor and Chair of Obstetrics and Gynecology, Division Head Maternal Fetal Medicine and Professor Molecular and Integrative Physiology at the University of Kansas School of Medicine, Kansas City, KS and the Crenshaw Professor and Chair of Obstetrics, Gynecology and Reproductive Biology, Division Head Maternal Fetal Medicine, and Professor of Physiology at the University of Maryland School of Medicine, Baltimore. Dr Weiner has published more than 265 peer-reviewed research articles and authored/edited 18 textbooks including *High-Risk Pregnancy: Management Options*. His research was extramurally funded for more than 30 years without interruption.

Professor Stephen Robson

Newcastle University, UK

Stephen C. Robson is Emeritus Professor of Fetal Medicine for the Population and Health Sciences Institute at The Medical School, Newcastle University. He is also a Consultant in Fetal Medicine for Newcastle upon Tyne Hospitals NHS Foundation Trust. He has published over 400 peer-reviewed articles and edited several; books, the highly successful being *High Risk Pregnancy: Management Options*. The fifth edition was published in 2018. He has been President of the British Maternal and Fetal Medicine.

About the Series

Most pregnancies are uncomplicated. However, for some ('high-risk' pregnancies) an adverse outcome for the mother and/or the baby is more likely. Each Element in the series covers a specific high-risk problem/condition in pregnancy. The risks of the condition will be listed followed by an evidence-based review of the management options. Once the series is complete, the Elements will be collated and printed in a sixth edition of *High-Risk Pregnancy: Management Options*.

Cambridge Elements ☰

High-Risk Pregnancy: Management Options

Elements in the Series

A full series listing is available at: www.cambridge.org/EHRP

Printed in the United States
by Baker & Taylor Publisher Services